YOUR BRAIN ON GLUTEN
(It's Not Just Celiac Disease)
Myths - Facts - Solutions

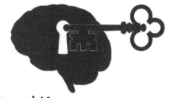

Jaqui Karr, cgp, csn, cvd

Dedicated to the misunderstood, misdiagnosed, mistreated.

You're *not* alone, and you *can* be well again.

"Please Keep Reading"

You'll probably want to tap out (more than once) as you read this book. Don't. For the love of your brain, body, quality of life in present and future - don't tap out.

When I first deep-dived into gluten research, 500-600 studies in, I realized what a complex spiderweb of a topic it is. Nothing is straightforward medically or legally:

-Test results aren't as simple as negative/positive and are inaccurate 69% of the time.

-Food labels that say gluten-free don't necessarily mean the food itself is gluten-free.

-Most stats are like mangled electrical wires, with no number being a true representation of the actual facts. Total mess.

It was (and still is) a complex spiderweb of information. I hadn't yet decided to turn all my professional focus on gluten, though everyone around me kept telling me not to. My own father: "You've suffered enough with this thing. I was having every parent's worst nightmare thinking I would have to bury my child. I thank God every day that you beat this. You're stronger than ever, now go back to the career you worked so hard to build and put this behind you."

I lied in bed that night thinking, *"But what about others? The system is set up for them to lose. I know I can help".*

There's only one place I go when I need to tap into source and get answers: The Ocean. I drove to Bar Harbor, Maine, and walked along the beach thinking about people I'd never meet. The condescending doctors' voices I first encountered were echoing in my ears: *"Your test results are more than fine, anti-depressants can take care of this self-induced anxiety."*

How many people wouldn't have my character to tell those doctors where they can put their prescriptions? How many of them would be defenseless children being put on ADHD medication and have no choice at all? How many more people would have their lives stolen from them, and what if I could intercept in some of those cases?

The right thing to do was clear, but I thought: *"How am I going to explain all this to others without holding them hostage for 20 hours and showing them facts they'd rather never see?"* (be warned if you ever sign up for one of my live seminars, but you can keep the handcuffs as party favors ;)

A decade later, this book takes that spiderweb of impossible data, along with the latest scientific updates, and lines it all up in a cohesive way for you. Just go slow. I promise, you'll want to tap out at certain points. Take breaks as needed, then come back. If you want the odds in your favor, *Please Keep Reading...*

-Jaqui Karr

Table of Contents

PART ONE: MOMENTS OF TRUTH

We'll start at the heart of the matter, expand to science, then return to the core for solutions. Have your highlighter handy, there are Power Tips throughout this entire book.

E.R. Moment of Truth

It was my 11th admission to the emergency room (13 in all, I had two more after diagnoses. I needed a few weeks to do damage control before I was off the I.V. forever).

...I'm in the corridor by myself, the rooms are reserved for wounded or trauma patients, *as they should be.* I was only there for 12 hours of I.V. to revive me before being sent back home. No tests this time, they were out of ideas. My mystery illness wasn't solved yet. No one could tell me why I kept fainting and why a sudden migraine chose to become a relentless, merciless monster, taking up permanent residence in my brain.

So far, MRI's, CAT scans, and all the other tests that had me five minutes away from glowing in the dark said it wasn't aneurysm, tumor, cancer, or MS. That's about all we knew. ...and that my blood tests were better than normal and I was in extraordinary health with perfect 7 pH levels. Great. I was bionically healthy, except for:

-A debilitating migraine that forced me to stop working, it was *literally* debilitating and created many bedridden days
-Fainting every 10-14 days, landing me in the E.R. (twice unconscious)
-30 pounds lost (from a 122-pound body)
-Unable to run for the first time in 24 years, some days unable to walk or get out of bed
-Clinically depressed, *on my best days*
-And I knew the ambulance drivers by first name, though I hadn't French kissed one yet, resuscitation hadn't made its way into the mix

...But the doctors and all the tests said I was perfectly fine, so I must have been perfectly fine. I wish someone had told me sooner what a phenomenal imagination I had, I could have given Walt Disney a run for his money. *(I tested for ways to cure the sarcasm, those tests came up empty too, they said it was incurable)*

Back to E.R. visit #11...

It was quiet. Midnight shift means minimum staff and it seemed the nurses and doctors weren't needed by any of the patients in the rooms of my corridor. One of those doors opened, ejecting a drug addict. I had seen the police bring him in, screaming and delirious, force-held down until a doctor injected a sedative. He had cracked his skull in an altercation and needed stitching. The bloodied bandages on his head told me they hadn't done this yet.

Next thing I knew, he flew through the air and landed on my gurney, climbing up my legs. I froze for a second, watching his blood zig-zag up my blanket. My first panicked thought was he wanted to rape me. He didn't. He wasn't after me, he was after the I.V. in my arm. He needed a fix and assumed there was more than saline in it. My hands were busy trying to keep him from ripping the needle out of my arm and ripping my skin apart, so the little red call button a few inches away from me may as well have been on a Tibet mountaintop.

No one was hearing my screams except me, they were ringing in my head through a nightmare I couldn't stop. I was at the back end of an L-shaped corridor, but it wasn't as long as a football field, someone should have heard me cry for help as I wrestled the crazed man. The man whose blood I could now feel on my bare arms, neck, face. Blood that was infected with... *I had no idea what.*

Someone finally did hear me, a janitor. He pulled the addict off me, and eventually more help arrived.

Deaf to the commotion of nurses and security as they contained the situation, I looked down at my purple arms. Four months of tests and I.V.'s created perpetually purple arms. One set of marks and bruises would barely heal before two more would replace it.

3:15 a.m., I had an E.R. Moment of Truth.

I realized I was facing death at the hands of the system. My previous visit had already found an infection dangerously close to my kidneys, serious enough to force me to take antibiotics, something I always thought should be avoided unless it's life and death. Well, the Grim Reaper was lurking in the shadows and drugs were now in my system.

I took the blood-stained gown off, leaving me with the yoga pants and t-shirt the paramedics brought me in with. I was unconscious for this one, so they were more rushed than usual and no one had stopped to grab my shoes or purse. December in Montreal, Canada, -22 Celsius (-7 Fahrenheit), the ground covered in ice, and I'm wearing the little blue paper shoes I stole from the E.R., along with a clean blanket from a shelf by the gurney, to act as a jacket.

Not wanting the cab driver to see me and suspect I was an escaped psyche patient, I took the long way around the parking lot so that I could get in from behind him. My plan was to get into my house using garage code, and hopefully my purse would be there so I could pay him. My feet were getting more and more numb with every icy step.

I jumped into the back seat within a second of opening the door and luckily, he was too startled from his nap to bother looking behind him. I made it home, without ever telling anyone at the hospital I left. I doubt anyone noticed or cared, their hands were full with bleeding patients. Mysterious invisible illnesses aren't their department (that's not sarcasm, just fact... E.R. isn't meant for chronic illness, it's meant for exactly what it's called: emergency).

In the longest shower of my life, I tried to wash away the night, the blood, the fear. Tears mixed with hot water, I stood under my rain shower and just cried. Into my bathrobe, I cried some more. Lit a fire, cried in front of it. Then I cried some more. And cried. And cried.

I'm not a crier, never have been. My mother used to poke me as a child to make sure I was still alive. I made up for a lifetime of not crying, all in one night.

And then I took charge. I didn't check out of the hospital officially, but now I did consciously officially check out of handing control over to doctors. I wrote a time line of everything that had happened, and then I made a tall press of java and waited for 8:30 a.m. The private clinic opened at 8:30. I was done with Medicare protocols, it was time for answers.

8:31 The receptionist said initial visits were 20 minutes. "Here's my American Express number, charge me for 40 minutes whether I use them or not, I need the doctor's undivided attention please. I need a double appointment please."

11:40 a.m. I sat in his office and held him hostage. My usually confident voice was quivering, which bothered me. I'm not used to feeling rattled and certainly not enough for it to come out in my voice. The poor man listened silently, but intently. He didn't interrupt me once, didn't look at me like I was crazy when I said it had to be a gut problem because migraine and depression have a common denominator and the gut is it, and hospital doctors said no, but I suspect they're wrong, and on and on I went. I talked in one continuous running sentence. I was scared that if I stopped for air, he might stop listening, like all the other doctors. He patiently listened and never interrupted.

Then I ran out of words, *and air.* He still waited silently a few seconds, looked at my tear-stained notes, and finally said: "I have an idea. Just sit right there, I'll be back in a few minutes." He was kind enough to not send me seven floors down to get a blood test. Instead, he brought a nurse up to me. My purple arms got one more jab.

3:20 p.m. the next day, I was back in his office. "Ms. Jaqui, a normal level of transglutaminase is under 10, you're at 44, do you know what Celiac Disease is? I'm sending you to gastroenterology for a biopsy."

Mystery solved, thanks to:
1) The drug addict in the E.R., I pray for his wellness.
2) The decision to take control, no matter how weak I felt.
3) A doctor who listened, and who had educated himself enough to know what Celiac Disease was. And more importantly, that its symptoms are neurological more often than gastrointestinal.

Enough about me, *Please Keep Reading...*

Don't let the word psychosis make you think it's an extreme and rare condition. You may fall into psychosis yourself when you realize how common brain issues are with gluten. Mild headaches and occasional brain fog, going all the way up to Alzheimer's and schizophrenia. You're probably somewhere in between, but don't let that scare you, this book is designed to get you on the right side of the tracks so that you can be solving complex crossword puzzles until you're 100 *(no promises at 101 ;)*

"Gluten Psychosis", the main title of a recent study. Even after a decade of intense studying and educating others on gluten, I still get the shock factor regularly. The moment I saw the title of that study, was the moment I decided to write this book.

The full title of the study is "Gluten Psychosis: Confirmation of a New Clinical Entity."[1] There's a part of me that wants to end this book right here, not sure if anything more needs to be said. If I didn't want to share solutions with you, this might have been a one-page book.

Gluten Psychosis. A New Clinical Entity.
A Psychosis Moment of Truth. *For all of us.*

Depression is actually the most common manifestation of gluten, but when I use the term "brain damage", know that it means everything from depression to dementia.

Brain damage caused by a food that has no unique nutritional value and is biologically unnecessary. *And we're eating it because...?????* ...Because massive corporations taught us to eat foods that have 50-year shelf lives so that they would have no waste, only profit. Those are the current tyrants.

If we rewind time, the tyrants before them realized grains were the cheapest way to keep slaves alive. The nobles (as they are now) were eating real food, while they were feeding grains to the slaves (that's you and me).

In between the two sets of tyrants were some well-meaning people, tired of being nomads and chasing food. I've lived enough Gypsy days to understand them. Grains provided the ability to settle down. Cohen said it well in one of his studies: "...we domesticated grain, and in return grain domesticated us."[2]

Good intentions, but it's time to correct the mistake, especially now that we have the ability to eat real food without needing to be nomads (though that would take care of another major problem, which is lack of movement).

I'm going to advise you to put a sticky note on your book or tablet as you read this book, with these two words: Keep Reading.

The challenge with science heavy books is: They're science heavy. Haven't we all had enough, *of everything?* Grim stats, nutrition this, food that, illness this, vitamin that, ... I've had enough.

My dream is to move to a surf village, ride waves every day, and sell seashell jewelry to put a roof over my head. I fantasize about never hearing the words gluten or disease again. I fantasize that perfect health is everyone's default state and no other states exist *insert deafening buzzer here* ...Hence this book, hence no seashell shop.

This book is equally about solutions as it is about making you aware of the magnitude of the problem, so hang in there when it gets heavy. I won't point out a single problem without also giving you the solution to it. I've got your back.

I know you don't really want to be reading this, and I wish I never needed to write it. I've put my seashell shop aside so that I can share with you what I've learned, because it matters. Because I care about you. Because I don't want you to find yourself in the dark stats a few years from now, or in the corridor of an emergency room with no answers.

Thank you for trusting me, I don't take this privilege and responsibility lightly. *Please Keep Reading...*

The Brain's Moment of Truth

Sometimes I'm not sure what to make of the way people malabsorb information. It makes me think of the stories of people who were raided by boats that they couldn't see, because it was something they couldn't understand or believe existed. *Big wooden things on the ocean, and they don't sink? Impossible.* Legend has it that Vikings and pirates cruised right up to their shores and they still couldn't see it. Not until their throats were being cut and it was too late.

When I tell people that "Gluten Sensitivity can be primarily and at times exclusively a neurological disease"[3], I feel like an invisible pirate ship. Everyone still thinks of nothing but bloated belly when you say gluten. I watch eyes glaze, but I know the stats, so I know the chances of that very person suffering from something they don't consider a brain problem. "Neurological Disease" sounds distant and severe. It's actually in the majority of homes: Depression, brain fog, ADHD, chronic sadness, mood swings, headaches, migraine, dementia... How many families do you know that are completely free of all of those things?

I came close to death with gluten damage and didn't have a single digestive symptom at first. All my issues were neurological, starting with a migraine, ending with severe depression. *Dangerous depression.* Those of you who have experienced it know what that means. If you're there now, hold on. You can still win this.

In between beginning and end, I had other neurological and nerve damage, one of which was: I started to lose feeling on my left side. EKG said no heart attack, MRI said not Multiple Sclerosis. Once again, I was told I was fine. Needing to walk with a walking stick told me I was *not* fine. I had been running 10 miles a day, on mountain terrain, just four months before the walking stick.

Tests and doctors said I was fine. I was *not* fine. And I was *not* receptive to their suggestions for pain medication and anti-depressants. That insane, barbaric approach needs to stop. Surely, there's another way for these people to make money without destroying people's souls.

There are children suffering seizures and being put on medication that sort of work. Many become non-responsive after a while and you already know the list of side effects... you've heard the sweet, calm, hypnotizing voice recite the (partial) list on TV ads while images of pretty flowers and butterflies enchant your eyes.

It's time to look at where those seizures are coming from and apply harmless solutions (like glutathione to repair the mitochondria so cells can talk to each other again instead of short-circuiting, a.k.a. seizures). ...That's just one example of a long list of fixable neurological problems. Hardly anyone is even trying these methods before going drug route.

This is the Brain's Moment of Truth. Our brains are in serious trouble and it's so outrageous, most people can't wrap their minds around the thought of their little slice of bread wreaking so much havoc.

The difference between my pirate ship and the Vikings' is that I won't be coming to shore, won't be raiding. I'll be anchored, solid in place, and it's up to you whether you choose to see the ship or not. I live and die by "Live and Let Live". I don't believe in force, even if it's for that person's best interest. I'll give you everything I've got: Knowledge, heart, soul. You choose how much of it you wish to see.

Please Keep Reading... (if your sticky note fell, find it, glue it back)

Nutritional Moment of Truth

We're at a crossroads as a collective society. We can continue what we've been doing the past 50-70 years as far as industrial food, and watch the complete collapse of humanity, or we can choose to stop at this point, with *only* 75% of the world sick (not just from gluten) and do what we can to reverse that number.

It's not about obesity versus beach body. It's about living with dignity, your mind intact to the end.

This entire book was inspired by the title of a study, but there are so many other study titles that leave me equally stunned. "Bread and Other Edible Agents of Mental Disease" found:

"... sciences of the facts that **bread**
1) **increases the permeability of the gut and likely of the blood-brain barrier in all of us**,
2) sets off an immune reaction in those of us who are genetically predisposed, and
3) breaks down, during digestion, in fragments with opioid activity"[4] (that's the equivalent of a heroin hit to your brain)

"Edible Agents of Mental Disease" needs a little more attention than it's getting. So does the fact that it causes gut damage in "all of us".

BREAD HOLDS NO UNIQUE NUTRITIONAL VALUE

Do we need bread from any nutritional standpoint? No. In fact, one of the top guys studying the gut and gluten specifically, says: "Gluten is, nutritionally speaking, useless."[5] He's not the only one. "No nutritional value has been attributed to gluten."[6]

People survived, disease-free, for millions of years, all gluten-free. And I can't help but point out: Totally raw for over a million years until fire was invented (not that I'm suggesting you become 100% raw, I'm just pointing out a fact). The remains of those people are the healthiest in history.

So why do we think we need gluten now? A handful of cereal-company-sponsored studies from the last year have been hitting the air waves about the importance of grains. They're failing to mention that breads and cereals wouldn't even have nutrients after 900-degree processing if they weren't synthetically enriched.

It's not just gluten and it's not just those with Celiac Disease. Wheat, overall, is a problem, as you'll see in a later chapter.

Grains, in general, are covered in lectins (wheat's being one of the worst). Lectins are the toxic poisons that protect a grain from being destroyed. It's a good poison, meant to keep the seeds alive so that the seeds can produce grass and feed us. Lectins are meant to keep away rodents, insects, mold, fungi. They do this by making critters anywhere from a little sick, to dead. Most rodents pick up the toxic scent and stay away. *...except human rodents, we keep eating...* Not only do we keep eating it, we keep coming up with new ways to use the food that's killing us. *We're engineering marvels.*

Every part of wheat, inside and out, is a problem for humans. Perhaps wheat grains were meant to keep providing nourishment in the form of wheat grass, which is one of the most powerful greens on the planet. Color Coded: Green is food, beige is meant to be grown into food. Notice that no fruit or vegetable is beige and dry. All healthy foods are colorful and high in water content.

Circle of life: You plant seeds, get more food.
Grind them down and eat those seeds: No more food.

We humans are so clever, we figured out a way to make infinite volumes of seeds. *Brilliant.* But we were never meant to eat them and they're killing us. So, what's our solution now? Add more human genius to the mix and make genetically modified, mutated, artificial, ninja wheat that has been engineered by biochemists and war biologists to make it through your digestive tract, regardless of what it does along the way.

We're at a Nutritional Moment of Truth.

Please Keep Reading...

Your Moment of Truth

You're reading this book, so obviously something is up. Hopefully not a major health crisis. Hopefully something reversible. Perhaps you're feeling a bit of a twitch when you have a lot of gluten and starting to realize that maybe you should investigate. Ultimately, you're in good shape and reading for knowledge, taking a preventative approach (congratulations on the progressive thinking). Or perhaps you're a health professional and want the hard facts.

The Marketing Masters tell me I'd sell more books if I told a lot of personal stories. They're fired. There's no time for stories, we passed the 11th hour three decades ago (not to mention, you've already been naked in the shower with me after I had my E.R. Moment of Truth, how do I get more personal than that?) I'm giving you a mountain of facts plus a mountain of solutions. I have faith in you. I have faith in your intelligence and ability to handle this information.

If your house was on fire, would you want the fireman to tell you a story, or throw a fireproof blanket over you and carry you to safety? I have news for you: Your house *is* on fire, it's called brain inflammation. I'm here to get you out, and it won't be over tea and crumpets. I might even bruise you a little, but you'll be safe from the fire, so forgive me for holding you extra tight.

Consider this Your Moment of Truth. It's the moment when you decide, before you keep reading, if you will silence all the media voices and cupcake-loving voices of fear, and just objectively look at the facts, and commit to reading to the end. *(GF cupcakes taste better anyways)*

I respect Your Moment of Truth, whatever road it leads you to. My singular job is to make sure you're making an informed decision. *Please Keep Reading...*

PART TWO: THE SCIENCE

You're going to think I'm giving you too much information. I'm not. When you find yourself in a conversation with several other people (or with an uninformed MD), outside your area of expertise and outnumbered, your mind will play tricks on you. I'm giving you enough information for that to never happen.

GLUTEN MYTHS

Fact versus Marketing Masters

Marketing sharp-shooters are good, they rarely miss their mark. Did you know some of the best copywriters in the world are paid $10,000 an hour and up? Some have a retainer fee of $75,000 just to have an initial consult. I know several personally and professionally.

Do you suppose they're paid that kind of money because they're ineffective? Do you think anyone would be insane enough to pay these guys and gals, and then invest millions of dollars in online ads to get your attention because there was no return on it and they just had money to burn?

Now team them up with trillion-dollar food makers and trillion-dollar pharmaceutical companies with unlimited budgets. What does that math add up to? The truth?

Marketing people can convince you that you were born from a different species if you give them enough of your attention. Convincing you a Gluten-Free Diet (GFD) is harmful is that much easier because you're already hard-wired to want to believe it (what's more primal than someone taking food out of your hands?)

This section shows you how media can muddy the waters and drown facts, sometimes completely unintentionally (doesn't make it less harmful). It's not just the marketing masters doing harm, it's also the people who are getting their gluten information strictly from online articles and then re-spinning the same flaws.

Look at the patterns here, and you'll know how to see clearly no matter what you read in the future.

Please Note: "Coeliac" (European, original spelling) versus "Celiac" (American spelling) are the same thing. I'm leaving them as is when I quote studies from around the world.

"It's Not Gluten, It's Glyphosate"

"It's not gluten, it's _____ *fill in the blank* _____", the biggest flavor of the month being Glyphosate. I can kill this demon in two minutes flat. Follow me please, into the history[7] of CD and we can put this Glyphosate issue to rest.

1st century AD: Greek physician Aretaeus of Cappadocia calls CD "Koiliakos", "suffering of the bowels" ("koelia" means abdomen). His notes have been translated and surprisingly passed on. His solution was to rest and fast, and if that didn't work, to purge. Fasting would alleviate the symptoms, I can see why he went that way. Problem is, as soon as the person picked up a piece of bread again... well, same problem as today. And you can't fast forever. Gluten Solution #1 (that we know of) was to stop eating entirely.

1793: Scottish physician and pathologist Dr. Matthew Baillie identifies textbook symptoms, noting diarrhea disappeared if patients ate only rice and no bread.

1888: English pediatrician Dr. Samuel Gee officially puts CD on the map by publishing "On the coeliac affection" (which quotes some of Aretaeus' observations and methods). Gee knew bread was the problem but hadn't zeroed in on the solution yet. CD is officially on the medical record and goes from "Koiliakos" to "Coeliac".

1908: Pediatrician Dr. Christian A. Herter publishes a book about Celiac Disease and children. He collaborates with Dr. Gee, in what gets referred to as Gee-Herter's Disease.

1924: U.S. pediatrician Dr. Sidney Haas and his "banana babies". His experiment of 10 Celiac children documented 8 that went on the banana diet improved while the 2 that continued eating bread died. *Died.* It's that serious even today. That paper did the rounds and thankfully helped some Celiacs live. Haas' Banana Diet excluded all cereals, breads, and potatoes. Still they hadn't isolated the issue to gluten, thinking it was all carbohydrates, but we're getting closer. *And eating bananas is an upgrade to fasting.*

...this is a good time to note that commercial pesticides and GMO's had not hit the market yet and we already had thousands of documented cases of CD across the world. CD was being studied in modern medicine since the late 1700's.

1944–45: Dutch famine, known as the Hongerwinter ("Hunger Winter"), a grain shortage as a result of a German blockade of food during WWII. Celiacs got better gluten-free. Post-war, grains became available again and the same patients got sick again. Now *there's* an unbiased unofficial study.

1952 Dutch pediatrician Dr. Willem Dicke introduces the Gluten Free Diet. *(Amen)*

...I'll stop the history lesson here, even though there were many more doctors, papers, and pegs on the gluten time line. I think the point is made?

1950's and on become "The Pesticide Era". Food, in general, begins to free-fall. No parachute in sight because the general public is unaware of the harm (70 years later, this is sadly still true).

1974: Glyphosate hits the commercial market by Monsanto under the name "Roundup". That's about 200 years after Celiac was being studied in modern medicine.

By the time Glyphosate or any pesticides hit the market, there were already tens of thousands of documented Celiac cases worldwide for almost 2 centuries, including the fact that they got better gluten-free, and sick again when they resumed eating gluten and grains in general. Those are modern medical records, the same as today's medicine, not mysterious hieroglyphics or ancient Greek.

I live and die by organic, so I would love to blame Glyphosate and its chemical brothers and sisters for all our gluten woes. As toxic as chemicals are for us, this time line irrefutably shows Glyphosate isn't the sole culprit because gluten damage existed long before any pesticides were even invented. *moment of silence for the death of that myth*

Chemicals accelerate and worsen the problem, it's yet another toxin our modern body has to deal with, so I'm not letting them off the hook. However, the point here is that Glyphosate-free or ancient gluten is still not good for you. For me. For anyone. It never was.

5 GENERATIONS OF MY FAMILY WITH "ANCIENT WHEAT"

I was born on ancient soil and ate old style bread made with ancient organic European wheat before moving to Canada. My mother hand-made bread, I still had issues. No Glyphosate in sight, only organic fermented bread.

At least five generations of my family all had major symptoms, the same as mine (note: no gastrointestinal issues at all). Predominantly eczema, dental issues, and neurological issues ranging from my mild headaches to my grandmother with suicidal depression...

"Mom, why do I get headaches and my friends at school don't?"

"It's genetic Honey. I've always had headaches, so did your grandmother - she had it the worst, your great-grandmother, and her mother..."

Genetic my @$$ *(sorry for my language Mom)*. My life-long headaches went away, forever, a few months after I was gluten free. The eczema went away in my 20's, I'm guessing because of how high raw and green I had become and it was counter-acting some of the effects of gluten. I still have eczema scars on my arms and legs, but I'm grateful the massive outbreak on the full left side of my face at age 9 didn't scar. My mom's home-made lotions and potions might have had something to do with that (Amen to cucumber mash preventing me from becoming the Phantomette of the Opera permanently). The kids at school had a field day with me. Makes me crazy that other kids are going through that this very moment...

In the decade I've been gluten-free at the time of this writing, I've had three restaurant contaminations, followed by weeks of migraine and then weeks of headache after that. It's instant and unquestionably a result of taking a gluten hit. Three consecutive, identical reactions. Thousands of others with Celiac Disease experience exactly the same.

Actually, not identical: I noticed it gets worse each time, so I did some cell memory research. It gets worse each time because your body is defending you. Celiac is a T-cell autoimmunity, but it's your B-cells[8] that remember the toxin from the last hit. Your body recognizes the enemy and builds a bigger and bigger defense each time. So if that happens to you, thank your body, it's doing its job. That "high alert" reaction can be scientifically measured and is shown to be 80% higher in those with Celiac Disease[9].

"It's not gluten, it's _____ _fill in the blank_ _____"

You can bet your life that you'll see many, many, many more things, like Glyphosate, blamed for illness in an attempt to exonerate gluten. It's an interesting (and heart-breaking) phenomenon to see how desperately people want to hold on to their regular burger bun and will readily accept any reason to do so while ignoring an overwhelming mountain of facts. _Indisputable facts._

Live and Let Live. I'm only here to present facts, do with them as you will, I respect your choices. The thing is: Absolutely every food you love can be made gluten-free. You don't give up what you love, you simply choose ingredients that are better for you. _Onward..._

"Higher Risks of Heart Disease on a GFD"

A 2017 study blazed the air waves and had the world convinced they would die of a heart attack if they went gluten-free.

Here's what the conclusion of the study actually said: "...the avoidance of gluten may result in reduced consumption of beneficial whole grains, which may affect cardiovascular risk. The promotion of gluten-free diets among people without celiac disease should not be encouraged."[10]

If you read the full study (no one ever does, not even doctors), they're talking about lack of fiber putting you at higher risk for heart disease, not lack of gluten.

Yes, we already knew the importance of fiber. But somehow, *can't imagine how* *cough cereal commercials* everyone decided it was a good idea to take a shortcut from the fiber in boring vegetables and get fiber from shiny boxes containing little plastic toys that are "enriched with fiber" (the plastic toy in its plastic wrapper is further toxifying our planet too, there's nothing good coming out of that box).

So, with convoluted modern-day logic, a group of scientists (who are on an average of three medications themselves), decided that "reduced consumption of beneficial whole grains may affect cardiovascular risk". No mention of the mighty broccoli anywhere in the study (I looked). Not a single tiny baby spinach leaf in sight (I double looked with a microscope and even sent in a green hound to sniff).

They didn't even study anyone, they studied data from other studies, designed for other purposes: "Consumption of gluten, estimated from food frequency questionnaires." The data was self-reported and "estimated", not measured in a controlled study. How accurate will you be if I ask you to give me a food diary of what you ate this past year? Year, not week.

It was a cohort study... *give me a few seconds of Geek Time please...*

Cohort means they study data and see if there are parallels. Which means we can make a link between the sun rising and Celiac Disease. The sun DID rise on the day that everyone with CD got diagnosed. I'm not being fresh *(ok, maybe a little)*, but that's how cohort studies work. They study data and make correlations. That can work if there's only one variable that changed, like a whole Amazon tribe, everything stays the same, add grains and they get sick, some die within a year (which has happened all over the world).

But you can't make a general link like fiber deficiency when there are hundreds of other variables that differ between study subjects and you never directly studied any of them. *Geek Time over.* That particular study: Useless and misleading.

NOTE TO SCIENTISTS PUBLISHING STUDIES: If you're going to publish a study regarding food and health, you might consider including real food, somewhere, *anywhere,* in the study as a comparison. Please study the gluten-free diet that's loaded with natural fiber from fresh fruits and vegetables, then report back to us. We'll be right here, chewing on raw carrots, waiting.
   -With love from Canada, not Russia, Jaqui Karr xo

SOLUTION: SOURCES OF FIBER FROM NON-SYNTHETIC, NON-PSYCHOSIS-INDUCING FOODS

   -Vegetables (Eat every vegetable you can find. Juicing doesn't count, you need it whole, which is why I'm giving you my secret weapon, dips and sauces, with several recipes and a better explanation in the NakedFood section. I wouldn't show you the problem without providing the solution)
   -Mushrooms (cloud ears higher in fiber, shiitake next)
   -Legumes
   -Lentils
   -Peas
   -Beans
   -Nuts
   -Seeds
   -Chia (fiber and clean omega-3's, recipes later)
   -Fruit (highest in persimmons, then apples, passion fruit, bananas, figs)
   -Flaxseed (don't let it sound boring, raw chocolate truffles are awesome, and no one will know they're made with ground flax)
   -Coconuts (the dehydrated slices make awesome snacks, travel easily, and are brilliant replacements to toxic potato chips... and here's the best part: eat as much of them as you want – try saying *that* with synthetic food)

"Higher Levels of Mercury and Arsenic in a GFD"

2017 was quite the year for muddy articles on the gluten free diet (I expect them to triple their quota of misleading articles in the next year). This one was designed to open the discussion regarding "The Unintended Consequences of a Gluten-free Diet".[11]

Here's what the study actually said: "While our study is cross-sectional and relies on self-reported data regarding gluten-free diets, it does suggest that future studies are needed to more fully examine exposure to toxic metals from consuming gluten-free foods."

It made no definitive statement, though that's all I saw on the Internet. Headlines should be legally mandated to carry at least 10% fact, at least when it comes to medical issues.

Here are the facts and why mercury and arsenic have even been brought up in a GFD...

MERCURY PART I

We know mercury is dangerously high in fish, but most don't know it's also found in High Fructose Corn Syrup (HFCS). If you examine products on the grocery store shelves that are gluten free, you'll find HFCS in almost every one of them.

Mercury disrupts your brain's metabolic process and alters neuronal plasticity. "Neurons lacking in plasticity are a factor in neurodevelopmental disorders such as autism and mental retardation."[12]

...You know that "convenient" breakfast you grab and go? 90% of them are loaded with HFCS/mercury and are promoting "mental retardation", which can mean brain fog and difficulty focusing, it doesn't mean you're running down the street naked chasing the mailman while barking (yet). *Good Morning.* I have a grab-and-go suggestion for you later that actually boosts your brain, improves memory, protects your precious neurons (and tastes better than the plasticized horrors labeled "nutritious"). It'll cost you 5 minutes a week to make it and bring your total grocery bill down.

Parents are loading their kids up on this stuff and then wondering why they're not doing well in school. *But the front of the box says "nutritious"!* Yes, and the front of my box says I'm still 22 years old. My driver's license says I'm 48. Read the ingredients list.

The question and answer to the mercury issue is: "What are people replacing gluten with?" Is it an organic banana or HFCS "health bars" laced with mercury?

MERCURY PART II

There's a non-food element to mercury that everyone has entirely missed, and that's the prevalence of dental decay being extremely high in those with Celiac Disease. High enough for the Michigan Dental Association[13] and Child Journal of Dentistry[14] to suggest that when dentists see unexplained dental decay in patients, they should immediately screen for Celiac.

That high prevalence often means years of dental work and metal fillings, pouring mercury into the person's bloodstream daily. As someone who was diagnosed with Celiac Disease later in life, sporting 21 root canals and 3 decades of unexplained, never-ending dental decay, I can personally attest to this matter. It took me years to replace all those fillings, and then a year of detox to clear the damage from my blood. Had I been in a study pre-detox, I would have only added to the myth that the cause is a gluten free diet. My silver fillings were the cause of high mercury in my blood, not my organic raw GF coconut flour cookie.

ARSENIC PART I

You'll notice a recurring theme, which is: "What are you replacing gluten with?" The two most common answers are corn and rice.

Rice naturally absorbs arsenic from soil and water. It's magnetized to it, more so than to any other grains. Remove wheat and replace it with rice daily, you might have an arsenic problem. However, if you replace the gluten with quinoa, chia, chick pea flour, coconut flour, almond flour... you avoid the problem (list of safe GF flours provided later).

...Bear with me on the biology lesson, this is so critical for your health, totally apart from gluten. It affects meat and vegetables, and becoming a problem in Paleo people too...

ARSENIC PART II

Arsenic is also present in non-organic meats. Many of the medications and feed given to animals is high in arsenic. High enough for the FDA to revoke approval from 3 out of 4 feed additives.[15]

That revoke status doesn't provide an immediate solution because producers are all allowed to deplete their existing stock before replacing it with approved products (which still contain toxins). Many producers have years' worth of stock remaining. While it would be a financial burden to dispose of this feed and replace it with less toxic ones, where does that leave the average consumer? Not a simple situation all around, but another source of arsenic, which obviously affects all meat eaters, not just people with CD.

ARSENIC PART III

Non-organic arsenic in soil is also naturally attracted to Sulphur, which is high in cruciferous vegetables. So, while someone might think they're doing a good thing eating more veggies, they might actually be poisoning themselves with arsenic. These include conventional broccoli, brussel sprouts, cauliflower, and kale (in my dreams the world replaces the word "conventional" with "toxic" ... *then I wake up*).

By the way, a few of those foods are on the famous "Clean 15" list. I'll rant about that list later. Drives me crazy when I see someone who's doing their best to make healthy choices but being given such bad guidance. By the time they get to me, they're exhausted, collapse into a chair, and say: "I don't know what else I can do, and I still don't feel well". After I dissect all their "healthy choices", my next challenge is to keep them from going postal.

SOLUTIONS

1) **Choose Organic.** Meats, vegetables, anything you consume. Forget the "Dirty Dozen and Clean 15". How does it make sense to eat "a little less poison"? It's still toxic and has a cumulative effect. I'm done with fatal baby steps, we need to grow up and be adults. Toxic is toxic, eat organic and stop giving yourself poison, at any level. You're getting plenty of poison from the air you breathe, car you drive... don't knowingly add to the list. There are plenty of things you have no control over, so do your best with everything you *do* have control over.

2) **Replace gluten with real food,** not highly processed products. If it doesn't expire within a week or two, it should raise an alert flag. Dehydrated and frozen may be exceptions, but examine the ingredient labels.

3) **Variety.** Corn and rice are inexpensive, abundant, easy for food manufacturers to rely on. Take a different route and explore varieties of foods that contain fantastic nutrients. Equally important is what they don't contain, which are some of the toxins discussed here.

"Weight Gain Caused by a GFD"

This myth was created to discourage the non-celiac people who are voluntarily choosing GF. 35% of several developed countries are voluntarily choosing GF. That's a huge financial hit for standard foods, so you can bet they're actively doing what they can to discourage it. It's the fastest growing market[16] in most developed countries. In the United States, 25% of adults said they were either decreasing or avoiding gluten completely.[17]

When I was first diagnosed, I was actually already 85% raw, though I never consciously thought of myself as "raw" at that time. Looking back, I was high-raw (defined by someone who is over 75% raw) since my early 20's.

But I did regularly eat gluten, thinking it was just a super-starch, never realizing the real damage it does. I thought since I worked out so much and had hard abs, I had nothing to worry about, it's not like it was sticking to my thighs. I wish I knew it was sticking to cell membranes in my brain, among other body parts.

Tuesdays were hand-made grilled red pepper calzone (Mi manchi Gianni), Friday nights were dedicated to wood-burning stove pizza with chianti, to honor Tuscany, where my pizza guru was from (Ti amo ancora don Antonio), and Sundays were Parisian croissants with triple espresso (Au revoir François). All hand-made from the best ingredients, with organic wheat (yet another myth).

Bidding farewell to my French baker and Italian chefs, I went to the grocery store. Forget higher risks of heart disease from untreated Celiac Disease[18], I had an instant heart attack from the ingredient labels of gluten-free foods. Thankfully, this has gotten slightly better since I was diagnosed, though plenty of terrifying GF foods are still on the shelves.

I found every variety of sugar I knew about and learned new names for sugars I didn't know existed yet. It was a challenge to find anything without High-Fructose Corn Syrup and all its cousins with funky names. Harmful fats, hydrogenated oils, artificial flavors, formaldehyde (we stain wood with that, don't know what it's doing in food), strange fillers I had to scientifically research to identify (when you take out the cheap wheat filler, you have to replace it with something... GF food is already higher in cost, it would be triple what it costs now without some kind of cheap filler, which is why raw food is even more expensive than GF food).

There were horrors on these labels that had me convinced I'd never fit in a sexy bikini again, just from reading the labels, not even eating the actual food-like substance inside those boxes.

POWER TIP: If you're newly diagnosed, before going to the gluten-free aisle, look for raw options for crackers, snacks, even breads. Breads might be harder to find, but raw crackers and snacks are popping up everywhere. You'll get the same crunch and texture you're looking for, more nutritious food, minus all the toxins and sugars. If you want to be a total super star, invest in a good dehydrator and take control of your food.

P.S. Don't get caught up in the stigma of "but I'm not a raw foodist". No one is saying you need to become one to grab a few awesome raw foods. You're not limited to the toxic GF aisle.

As far as GF and weight gain, I don't need to cite a medical study on this one... Yes, going gluten-free can cause weight gain...

The beach-body-killing question is: When someone removes gluten from their diet, what do they replace it with? All too often it's not organic, real food, but highly processed, sugar and harmful-fat loaded food that even a triathlete couldn't stay thin on.

Of course you'll gain weight if you double your sugar and toxin intake. Tradesmen wear oxygen masks to avoid inhaling formaldehyde, and it's in several processed GF foods I've seen. Do you suppose that's causing thyroid, hormonal, organ malfunction?

I can't believe the things that get air time on the Internet.

"Celiac Disease is a Fad"

...that's one hell of a fad that stood the test of time... As fear grows, so does denial. It started out as the gluten-free diet was a fad, and now I'm starting to hear Celiac itself is a fad, "doesn't exist, it's just the pesticides, fructans, _____*fill in the blank*_____".

1888 "On the coeliac affection"[19]

1923 "Two Cases of Cœliac Infantilism in the Convalescent (Non-diarrhœic) Stage"[20]

1924 "DISCUSS ON SPRUE AND COELIAC DISEASE"[21]

1925 "A Case of Cœliac Disease with Glycosuria"[22]

1927 "The Bone Changes Occurring in Renal and Coeliac Infantilism and their Relationship to Rickets"[23]

1927 "A Note on Gluteal Wasting as a Sign of Cœliac Disease"[24]

1928 "Coeliac Disease"[25]

1929 "Chronic Intestinal Indigestion (Coeliac Disease)"[26]

1933 "Studies in the Anæmias of Infancy and Early Childhood: Part III. The anhæmatopoietic anæmias (deficiency diseases of the erythron): nutritional anæmia, and the anæmias of prematurity, scurvy and cœliac disease"[27]

A hundred years, millions of patients, and 40,000+ studies later, the spelling has changed slightly, the attitude has barely moved an inch.

The saddest part isn't that CD is being called a fad by the fearful public, it's that within the medical system, many of the same issues from a hundred years ago are still mis-diagnosed.

1927 they wrote on "gluteal wasting". 1972 Paris studied "Anorexic forms of celiac syndromes."[28] In the new millennium, people with severe anorexia or bulimia are still misdiagnosed as mentally ill patients and given anti-depressants instead of being screened for gluten antibodies or CD. Even with a study of this magnitude, the medical system is still not making the connection:

"18 000 women with celiac disease (CD) showed a positive association between CD and anorexia nervosa (AN) both before and after CD diagnosis... The bidirectional association between AN diagnosis and CD warrants attention in the initial assessment and follow-up of these conditions because underdiagnosis and misdiagnosis of these disorders likely cause protracted and unnecessary morbidity."[29]

...unnecessary morbidity indeed...

"Neurological disorders and adult coeliac disease."[30] That was 50 years ago, yet the connection of gluten to brain disorder is only now being "discovered".

We're writing new medical papers to celebrate anniversaries...

"Coeliac disease: one century after Samuel Gee (1888)."[31] *Happy 100,* but we're still not getting it right. Maybe at the 200-year mark. On the record: if I re-incarnate as a health-conscious person, you're on your own, I'm going to be a professional surfer next time around! They better have gluten figured out by then.

Fad. Good Grief. *another moment of silence for the death of that myth*

"We've Been Eating Wheat for 10,000 Years"

Actually, 20,000, it's just 10,000 since domesticating it, and the challenge with that statement is that it implies we've been eating wheat with no problem. That's not what the facts say. The facts say that every time wheat is introduced to a society, a very consistent number of things happen: Tooth decay, bone loss, iron deficiency, anemia, shorter stature (by 3-5 inches), obesity, disease (too many types to list, both body and brain), and higher mortality rates. The bones of our faces actually shrink, which is what causes crooked/crowded teeth[32].

While we've definitely been making a bad thing worse with modern wheat, and we can sit here and analyze 200 peptides within wheat, go beyond basic gliadin, scrutinize how the Glia-α9 epitope might be playing a factor in higher levels of Celiac Disease in the past few decades...[33] At the end of the day, what we started out with 20,000 years ago wasn't good for us either.

In the grand scheme of things, we haven't been eating wheat that long. 20,000 divided by 2,500,000 years we ate pure food = 0.008 of our existence.

It's going to seem like I'm digressing with the next few paragraphs, but I'm not. I'm going to use an example to give you a 30,000-foot view of what happens on the topic of gluten constantly. See how easily the facts get buried under statements with zero basis, and why you're programmed to accept it (not your fault). This is only one example, stay with me and it'll make sense in a minute...

I've mentioned gluten and dental issues a few times. Well, here's one of those times when our Hollywood-dependent culture creates wires crossing in our brains when we face real data.

Before eating grains/wheat: The real data, based on archaeological findings (bones don't lie), say that we used to have no dental decay. We had overall better bone density throughout our body.
"Prehistoric dental treatments were extremely rare, and the few documented cases are known from the Neolithic, when the adoption of early farming culture caused an increase of carious lesions."[34]

After eating grains: 16-49% dental decay on teeth recovered.[35]

Q: Can it be some other factor we're unaware of? How do we know it's wheat?

A: Because modern day cultures that don't eat grains have less than 1% dental decay. Introduce grains and they have dental issues within a few short years. Take grains away and the issues decrease again.

Dr. Weston Price was a dentist who was so baffled by how much dental decay he saw, he quit his practice, and traveled the world (1930) to investigate if nutrition was involved. In 1939 he published "Nutrition and Physical Degeneration"[36], pointing dental decay primarily to flour, sugar, processed fats.

So, if cave people had great teeth, why do we all have the impression they had bad teeth?

When you see caveman movies, you don't see the picture of health, do you. You see toothless, dirty, scruffy, scraggly-haired beasts that have lice and other creatures on their head. You can almost smell their awful body odor through your television screen. Roman gladiators, on the other hand, women might be tempted to give up their firstborns for.

Those toothless cavemen in movies are not what archaeologists have found. The hard proof is showing us they had fantastically healthy, straight teeth and much better overall bone health than we do. Their women weren't plagued with osteoporosis like ours are. So, why is osteoporosis and dental decay rampant if we're so smart and advanced (I paid over $200 for my last toothbrush), when it didn't exist in caveman days, when they weren't paying attention to any of it. Goodness knows they weren't taking calcium supplements.

By the way, the sexy gladiators... they were eating grains, had dental issues, digestive issues, inflamed colons, depressed, had lower bone density, and were 5 inches shorter than cavemen. Sorry to break the image.

But notice how Conan the Barbarian was ultra-sexy and had a wonderful set of straight sparkling white teeth, moisturized skin, healthy shiny hair, and a glistening hairless body (did razors exist back then?) I can practically smell the cologne. So why isn't *that* our overall impression of cavemen? Because for every 1 Conan, there are 10,000 toothless ape-like hairy beasts. Repetition creates perception, and perception becomes reality.

We can't blame Hollywood for entertaining us, we pay them to entertain us. Their job is to entertain, not educate. But if we're relying on Hollywood for history lessons and education...

Do you remember when comedian Jon Stewart got put under scrutiny for a while for his "obligation" in reporting political news? Absolutely insane. I remember seeing him on CNN (best thing I ever saw on CNN, where he brilliantly, effortlessly, clobbered the useless so-called journalists, I don't know how those two ever showed their faces again) and I'm paraphrasing: "Hey guys, I'm on the Comedy Network and come after a Muppets show".

I didn't tell you this to go off on an entertainment tangent, there's actually an important purpose. I want to point out that sometimes when we're facing real facts, it can be easy for our brain to unconsciously reject it, because we've had conditioning from so many sources, including unintentionally from movies. I'm positive no movie producer had gluten on their mind when toothless cavemen were depicted, but they set a very heavy impression on the world of what cavemen supposedly looked like.

That's Hollywood conditioning. How are devout Catholics supposed to reject the "daily bread" that they've been praying to their God for every day since being in the womb and listening to their mothers pray? (Did you see my rant online when the Pope declared GF communion was unapproved by the Vatican? The only time I've ever made a statement regarding religion. *Any* religion.) That's powerful opposition for hard core believers. Several Catholic Celiacs commented on that thread and said they felt conflicted. ...I would think the Pope would have better things to do and not jump on the GF bandwagon too, but I've learned that even amoebas use their single cell to write articles about gluten.

In Morocco, bread is so holy, you can't even apply a knife to it, you can only break it with your hands. The name for bread is the same word as for "life" and present at almost every meal. Care to know the higher prevalence of schizophrenia in Moroccans? (that question will become more significant in the coming chapters, bank it) The Netherlands actually compared the rates of schizophrenia of Moroccan migrants to their native Dutch population and found double the incidence.[37] How do we fit *that* fact into a sexy Hollywood movie? And how do you tell a Moroccan that their sacred "life" bread may be the reason they suffer higher rates of dementia?

Now that you're aware, when you feel that resistance as you see facts, that little part of you that says *"it can't be"*, you need to consciously step into the picture and realize that one of two things are happening:

1) You wish it wasn't true, so you're looking for a way to reject the facts (we tend to do this with bad relationships too).

2) There's so much mental conditioning, a lifetime of media programming, even cultural and religious programming, that it's creating a mental disconnect from the data in front of you. You have to find a way to over-ride the mental conditioning.

GLUTEN FACTS

The Celiac Spectrum

Needless to say, I had some challenging moments when Celiac put itself on my dance card. Of many things that happened, *even the bleeding addict trying to rip the I.V. out of my arm,* nothing got me outraged. Annoyed, frustrated, apprehensive, scared, discouraged, depressed, but never outraged. Using the word outrage is almost like using the word hate, you need to consider if you truly feel that strongly.

Here's what got me outraged about Celiac Disease: How the medical system officially diagnoses it. *...I know,* you were expecting something more dramatic. Hang in there, it'll make sense in a minute.

"The Marsh Method" is based on intestinal biopsy and it's still the standard of how CD is diagnosed.[38] They insert a tube down your throat, take 2-3 swabs —I have to stop right here and point something out:
--They take 2 or 3 little swabs from the very top end of 22 feet of intestines. That alone is an issue, since the intestines don't get damaged evenly in all spots--
...and with those swabs, which are less than a 0.0001% sample, they determine what level of damage your intestines are at. It's measured as 0 (no damage), then 1, 2, 3, 4.
The final stage, 4, is called "total villous atrophy", which is the medical equivalent of "total devastation". The word atrophy is used for more than intestines. It's when some part of your body gets diminished, whether it's muscle, brain, tissue... anything. It could be mild, right up to debilitating or fatal.
If your biopsy shows you're at stage 0-3, the pathologist will write "negative" on your file and depending on how your doctor's office communicates with you, you might never be the wiser. Many doctors' offices don't call you in unless there's a positive diagnosis. So, like hundreds of people I've met, and thousands more I've read about, the receptionist will call and say "Nope, negative on Celiac, you're fine to eat anything you want."
...The atrophy will continue...

Now imagine we did that with cancer: "You're only at stage 3 cancer, don't worry about a thing, it's negative. Come back in 2-3 years for another biopsy and we'll see if it's at stage 4 yet, and then you can start doing something about it."

Can you imagine the outrage? There would be protests and marches in the streets. Can you imagine the lawsuits? The number of preventable deaths? The number of people with a treatable health issue that was easy to reverse and now has gone too far to heal... We do this with Celiac Disease all day, every day, all over the world.

Note: Most doctors are still using the standard Marsh Method. There's also something called the Modified Marsh Method, which takes 0-4 and relabels it as 0, 1, 2, 3a, 3b, 3c, with 3b putting up a yellow flag and 3c replacing the 4. Same difference. Same issue of taking a few swabs from 22 feet. Same lack of timely warnings. Same levels of misdiagnoses. Same unnecessary time lapse/health deterioration until correct diagnoses. And not everyone affected gets intestinal damage, we'll get to that in a minute.

WHY THEY WON'T DIAGNOSE BEFORE STAGE 4

Since they're not here to defend themselves, I'll clarify why the system is set up as it is. The reason they warn you with cancer and not with Celiac is because with cancer, it's almost guaranteed to get worse and become fatal. With Celiac, some people can remain in stages 0-3 and never get to 4, so the medical system doesn't want to cause "unnecessary alarm".

Issues with that approach:

1) Serious, even fatal issues still happen in stages 0-3 of CD, as you'll see throughout this book. You're also more likely to trigger multiple other disorders while your system continues to get weaker, many of them are irreversible.

2) The patient has a right to know and I believe it's their doctor's responsibility to be knowledgeable and explain all the potential risks, even if there's no way to know whether stage 4 will happen or not. I shouldn't be explaining it in a book, your doctor should be explaining it in their office.

Who is telling the children who just lost their young mother, *"Well, chances were she wouldn't die, so we don't warn. Everything is fine, keep shopping and keep eating pizza."* ?!?!?

And what about millions suffering from unexplained depression? *"You've been fighting depression all your life, your blood is drowning in antibodies, your brain cells are dying in the glycation process from gluten, but you have no intestinal damage we can see, it doesn't matter if the depression goes away GF, the medical book says you're not a Celiac, keep eating gluten because it's a healthy whole grain, like the government says."*

3) NCGS means no intestinal damage and no Celiac genes, which would put you *nowhere* on the map as far as standard testing goes. But it doesn't mean no antibodies, gluten-related inflammation, depression, arthritis, nerve damage, brain damage... Throughout this book I'll show you studies of severe health issues (including dementia) with patients that have zero intestinal damage but a whole lot of antibodies to gluten. Given that fact, even stage 0 becomes irrelevant.

The medical data says 2/3 of the time the cause of neuro damage goes under the radar because there are no gastro symptoms.[39] So, we know there are no gastro symptoms most of the time, and the only way we determine CD is by measuring intestinal damage... we're *knowingly* failing all those people. Millions of people.

Even if your intestines are fine for now, would you want to know if you have antibodies that people with Alzheimer's have in your blood, making dementia much more probable for you? Would you want to know your food habits are creating an 8 times higher risk of premature death with liver disease[40]?

Are you outraged? Would you be outraged if you were at stage 3 on the spectrum, for *any* disease, and sent home and told you're fine?

"Complicated coeliac disease is an extremely serious condition with a high mortality and a short survival."[41]

It Was Never 1%

Now that you understand The Celiac Spectrum and how testing is ignoring the majority of people on the spectrum, you'll understand several more elements, starting with why it's grossly incorrect to say that only 1% have Celiac Disease. Get your calculator ready...

ONLY 1 OUT OF 9 ARE DIAGNOSED

Gut[42] and Gastroenterology[43] journals have already stated that for every 1 diagnosed, 8 are not. That one fact, by itself, obliterates the 1% myth. In the U.S. alone, that jumps the number of people with (biopsy diagnosable) Celiac from 3.2 million to 30 million. *Keep adding...*

1 IN 9 COUNTS ONLY STAGE 4

The 1 in 9 is referring ONLY to people officially diagnosed by biopsy and at stage 4. They're not referring to people who are in stages 0, 1, 2, 3 - and the total number of people in those stages is obviously the bigger number. We know there are more people in earlier stages because the average Celiac goes 11-17[44] years undiagnosed, according to the medical records on both sides of the ocean. "Every time the disease is clinically diagnosed in an adult, that person has for decades had disease in a latent or silent stage."[45] *Keep adding...*

35-40% HAVE THE GENES FOR CD

Over 35% of the population have the genes for Celiac Disease[46] with only one exception: The Japanese.

That doesn't make them exempt from NCGS or wheat allergy, they just don't have the genes for CD. Don't let that fool you into thinking the Japanese get away with muffin festivals unscathed. Gluten hits their brain hard too: "Gluten sensitivity is involved in at least some of the unexplained neurological symptoms of Japanese patients with adult-onset, sporadic cerebellar ataxia."[47]

No one on earth is escaping gluten effects.

Now here's an un-scientific question for you, I'd love to know your opinion: When gluten is causing brain injury (cerebellar ataxia) which could lead to seizures, involuntary movements, paralysis, and even death if the brain inflammation advances too fast for trauma doctors to drain it, do you really need an official Celiac diagnosis to stop eating gluten? (As I ask that question, millions of Homer Simpsons are saying "Mmmmm, donut"). Back to the Celiac genes...

Over 35% of people in most countries are somewhere on the Celiac Spectrum, like ticking time bombs, suffering minor and major symptoms that they think are either normal or they've been misdiagnosed and being incorrectly treated for something else (depression, ADHD, full range of neurological disorders, IBS, Hashimoto's are most common).

"Celiac disease is often missed since not only are clinical findings 'not typical' but also because many cases are asymptomatic."[48]

No symptoms + hundreds of different manifestations = it gets missed often. How's your calculator doing? *Keep adding...*

7% WITH CELIAC DISEASE DON'T HAVE THE GENES

The complex spiderweb gets a few more spins...

Up until recently, we thought it was an absolute that you had to have one or both genes to have Celiac Disease. Not so. A recent study did blood work on biopsy-confirmed Celiacs and found 7% of them didn't have either of the genes.

Finland had also done a study[49], finding the genes missing in 5% of their Celiac subjects.

5%. 7%. There's no way to know the exact number until very large-scale studies are done. The only thing we can be certain of is that not everyone with CD has the genes for it (maybe there are more genes we haven't discovered yet). This means that besides NCGS, which "We do know that the number of individuals with gluten sensitivity is exploding"[50], we also need to add a new set of people who are officially diagnosed with CD, who don't have the genes, on top of the 35-40% who do have the genes.

I'm not trying to guess what the total number is. I don't believe in guess work. However, we know beyond any doubt that the number is obscenely higher than 1%.

It was 2003 when the medical system itself said: "Celiac Disease is a much greater problem in the U.S. than has previously been appreciated"[51] (every country has issued the same statement), but since we can't quantify the number, everyone is going along with status quo. I've always said maybe they just printed too many t-shirts that said "1 in 133" and they didn't want to waste them. *(Car washes need spare rags all the time folks, give up the 1 in 133 number already)*

We're still not done. *Keep adding...*

ADD 6X FOR NCGS + WA

So far, we've counted only official Celiac Disease via gene susceptibility or biopsy. Now we need to add Non-Celiac Gluten Sensitivity (6 times more prevalent than CD) and Wheat Allergy, which are separate entities of their own. What number are we at?

The number of people affected is NOT 1%. It was never 1%.

"The association between gluten related disorders and psychiatric diseases has been firmly demonstrated. Non-celiac gluten sensitivity (NCGS) is a syndrome diagnosed in patients responsive to gluten-free diet after ruling out celiac disease and wheat allergy."[52]

The NCGS Brain

The last chapter showed you that the Celiac 1% myth is SO far off the charts, that at present, there's no way to even calculate how many of the susceptible 35-40% (with genes) + 5-7% (without genes), *all somewhere on the spectrum,* should be considered as living with Celiac Disease (Shouldn't they all? Isn't a bomb still called a bomb, regardless of when or if it's going to go off?)

Now we add NCGS to that number, "gluten sensitivity (GS), has emerged as an illness distinct from celiac disease with an estimated prevalence **6 times that of CD** ...gluten sensitivity remains undertreated and underrecognized as a contributing factor to psychiatric and neurologic manifestations."[53]

NCGS 6 times more prevalent than Celiac Disease and does brain damage too. What percentage of the population are we up to, with conditions we can immediately diagnose, never mind the things still brewing below surface that won't pop up for a few years? *Or months. Or days.* I ran a 26-kilometer marathon 6 weeks before my first E.R. visit. I know first-hand that the bomb can go off anytime.

NCGS isn't just more common, it's more deadly: Risk of premature death 39% higher with CD and a whopping 72% higher with NCGS.[54] As far as premature death goes, people should be twice as concerned with NCGS than with CD.

The current data, with the latest technology in testing, is showing definite neurological disorders affecting both Celiac and Non-Celiac patients[55]. It's hitting the person who is predisposed to Celiac with not just minor inflammation, but transforming them to a "hyperexcitable celiac brain"[56]. Picture dynamite with a long ignition string leading to it. Gluten is the match. Set a match to the ignition, the fire crawls up the string (the human spinal cord), and shoots to the brain, disconnecting things along the way (seizures, numbness, brain fog...).

It's hitting the brain of non-Celiacs just as hard, full range from mood disorders right up to schizophrenia.[57] That's the same as fatal in my eyes. What kind of life do you have if you're schizophrenic?

This is one of those moments I usually pace my living room or go for a walk outside because I can't believe what I'm writing. I have the studies stacked in a pile in front of me, and it's still surreal to me, so I can only imagine what you're thinking, thank you for staying. *Please Keep Reading...*

THE NCGS BRAIN (from the same paper quoted above, I won't even dive into my pile to bring on additional studies)

-Attention deficit hyperactivity disorder (ADHD)
-Autism spectrum disorders
-Depressive and mood disorders
-Epilepsy and Seizure Disorders
-Gluten Ataxia
-Headache
-Inflammatory myopathies
-Myelopathies
-Peripheral neuropathy
-Schizophrenia
-Social phobia and panic disorder
-Gluten encephalopathy

MEDICAL JARGON BLINDS US

"Gluten encephalopathy" makes it sound like some extremely rare form of disease in a faraway land. It just means brain damage from a toxin. Your mild headaches can be classified as gluten encephalopathy, so can severe dementia.

"Patient with Gluten Encephalopathy Presenting with Neuropsychiatric Symptoms."[58] ...*4 corners of the earth*, that one is Pakistan.

Gluten encephalopathy again, this time Italy: "After worsening of his neuropsychiatric conditions, with the onset of a frontal cognitive deficit, bradykinesia and difficulty walking, dysphagia, anorexia and hypoferraemic anaemia."[59] The patient went into full remission of all symptoms after going gluten free, and they diagnosed her with only anti-gliadin antibodies, not biopsy.

Effectively, all brain disorders can fall under the encephalopathy umbrella. By separating the disorders, we lose sight of how many people are affected. They do the same with autoimmune disorders in general, they break it down into so many categories and different disease names, that no one realizes over 24,000,000 people in the U.S. alone have been diagnosed with an autoimmune disorder[60] (bigger problem than heart disease).

Don't allow the terms and way the stats are reported blind you, gluten is a serious epidemic worldwide, with severe and fatal consequences, mostly affecting the brain.

HOW LONG SHALL WE KEEP CALLING IT UNKNOWN ORIGIN?

The data says that about 22% of people with Celiac develop neurologic or psychiatric dysfunction[61] and 57% of people with brain disorders of "unknown origin" test positive for anti-gliadin antibodies[62].

57%. The majority of people with mysterious brain disorders have gluten antibodies in their blood. Seems kind of significant, don't you think?

"Current medical practice leaves a significant proportion of these cases undiagnosed."[63] At least there's no favoritism, NCGS is being ignored as much as CD.

Exotic mosquitoes and flees are getting more air time than gluten, and I've never known any mosquito bite to put people in psyche wards. 100+ years of a particular flee putting tens of thousands of people in psyche wards would create a worldwide manhunt for that flee, with scientists scrambling to find an antidote. They would figure out how to turn back time and obliterate the first two from Noah's Ark.

All we need to do is replace gluten with one of a hundred other options, and we're resisting this solution? Maybe it's my "hyperexcitable" Celiac brain, but I can't make sense of it.

"GLUTEN SENSITIVE" STARTING TO INCLUDE CD AND NCGS

Many of the newer studies aren't bothering to differentiate Celiac from NCGS anymore. They're starting to refer to both groups as "Gluten Sensitive" (GS), because the end effects and *co-morbidity are the same. (*co-morbidity means other disorders created from one disorder, in this case gluten related disorders)

"...all patients with diagnosis of undifferentiated connective tissue disease, especially those with a systemic sclerosis-like presentation, should be investigated for celiac disease, even in absence of gastrointestinal symptoms. Gluten-free diet should be early recommended to all patients having undifferentiated connective tissue disease and gluten sensitivity."[64]

After examining biopsies from Celiac and NCGS patients, they're finding that with certain neurological issues, like gluten ataxia, it "is better classified as non-celiac gluten sensitivity than as celiac disease."[65]

Gluten ataxia, Alzheimer's, dementia, cognitive impairment[66] with NCGS. Zero intestinal damage. That means that by the medical system's own data, the way we currently test is useless 60-70% of the time. I don't say this to rant or criticize, I'm aware it's not easy to update medical books. I'm telling you this to make you aware of where you stand versus where the system is for now, and where it will be for decades. Medical books are updated every 30-40 years. *Informed Decisions.*

"The "psychomicrobiotic": Targeting microbiota in major psychiatric disorders..."[67]

Our health crisis is creating interesting new terms. "Psycho-microbiotic". Well, at least the connection is being made between gut health and brain / emotional health. ...it was in ancient hieroglyphics, but it's still nice to see it being "discovered" now...

Gluten and Your Gut (100% of the Population)

This study needs to be all over the media instead of the latest athlete or actor who has gone gluten-free:

"...gliadin exposure induces an increase in intestinal permeability in all individuals, regardless of whether or not they have celiac disease."[68]

All individuals get gut damage from gluten, including:
-Celiac Disease
-NCGS
-Wheat Allergic and Non-Wheat Allergic
-And "normal", meaning none of the above

ALL, 100% of them, reacted negatively 30-120 minutes after eating gluten. That's awfully fast. And it's ongoing. It's like unleashing an army of evil ants (gluten antibodies) into your body and those damn things crawl everywhere for months.

Something to clarify: You'll hear the word "gliadin" as if there's only one. There are over 200 (that we know of so far) and the human body can't digest *any* of them.[69] [gliadins are prolamin, a class of proteins]

...We're one minute in and already need a summary:
1) The human body can't digest any of the 200+ gliadins in wheat
2) Gluten causes gut damage (intestinal permeability) in all humans

INTESTINAL PERMEABILITY, MEDICAL DEFINITION

Also called Leaky Gut Syndrome (LGS)
"Gastrointestinal tract dysfunction caused by antibiotics, toxins, poor diet, parasites or infections, leading to increased intestinal wall permeability and absorption of toxins, bacteria, fungi, parasites, etc; LGS may be linked to allergy and autoimmunity"[70]

In layman's terms: It creates holes in your gut and allows bad things to penetrate your body, which leaves you susceptible to various medical issues. Gluten breaks down your natural fortress and puts you in a weak position. The direct damage gluten is doing is one thing, but all the potential effects are where we get into even more trouble, and that is trouble that's not easy to identify or link back to cause. Dangerous mushroom effect.

MAJOR DEPRESSIVE DISORDER AND LEAKY GUT

We know gluten causes leaky gut in everyone, Celiac/NCGS or not. This study linked major depressive disorder (MDD) to leaky gut. They weren't testing for gluten or Celiac specifically. Their entire focus was depression and leaky gut: "There is now evidence that major depression (MDD) is accompanied by an activation of the inflammatory response system... patients with MDD should be checked for leaky gut by means of the IgM and IgA panel used in the present study and accordingly should be treated for leaky gut."[71]

MOST PEOPLE ARE ASYMPTOMATIC

I repeat for good reason: Most patients show no symptoms. ...or at least like me, plenty of symptoms if you know what you're looking for, but we've taught ourselves that those things are normal or hereditary. Think about what the world accepts as normal...

Indigestion. How many tons of pink stuff and antacids and food digestion or heartburn pills does the developed world consume in a year? *How can that possibly be normal??* How can we possibly be conditioned to think we need synthetic help to eat synthetic food? Why wouldn't we stick to food our bodies know how to process?

Skin Issues. How many tons of cortisone ointment are prescribed per year? Prescriptions without any effort to find the cause of these calls for help the body is sending out. Meanwhile, they call dermatitis herpetiformus[72] (itchy swelling skin issue) the sister disease to Celiac.

Again, erasing the line between CD and NCGS, and referring to both groups with the term Gluten Sensitivity: "Dermatitis herpetiformis is currently regarded as the skin manifestation of gluten sensitivity."[73]

Thousands of cases of eczema[74], psoriasis[75], this skin disorder list goes on... and they all usually go into full remission gluten free.[76] *Yet the cortisone keeps flowing from the Pharma Infinity Fountain of Cream and is the only solution in most doctors' offices.* I was 9 years old when I told my mom no more creams, they were futile and did nothing but add a bad smell to my life. I eased cracked feet by soaking in warm water and cooled itching elbows and knees with cool cloths. *That's not normal,* yet it got passed off as normal for my entire childhood and teens.

DERMATITIS, ECZEMA, PSORIASIS

Besides the fact that they *almost always go away GF, it's important to note that when these skin issues are severe, they're creating lesions. Your skin is there to protect you from environmental toxins. When there are cuts (the same as open wounds), you're now that much more vulnerable to yet even more issues.

So much attention is put on the blood-brain barrier or toxins getting through a leaky gut. One step faster than both of those is toxins getting into your system right through your open skin. "Some studies indicate increased prevalence of cancer in patients with psoriasis, probably due to negative influence of skin lesion."[77] Psoriasis sufferers often have gluten antibodies (antigliadin IgA) in their system.[78]

*Note: I say "almost" always go away GF because sometimes there's extensive damage that requires deep, clinical level detox. Once this is done, and GFD is maintained, the more stubborn cases can also find relief of symptoms. Also, symptom relief can be as fast as a few weeks with eczema or mild skin issues, but often take longer (9-14 months) with psoriasis and more severe issues. People will often try a few weeks, not see results, and quit. We're talking cell damage and worse, it can take longer than a few weeks to detox, heal, and renew.

We tend to dismiss things like skin issues, not treating them as serious health issues (like they did with me as a kid). "A number of studies suggest that psoriasis and celiac disease share common genetic and inflammatory pathways."[79] Perhaps psoriasis shouldn't be classified strictly as a dermatological issue but also a deadly inflammatory disease and an autoimmune response. Perhaps with more serious classifications, the root cause would seem more important and we wouldn't be dismissing these skin issues with topical creams.

Forget Celiac Disease, that's only one manifestation of gluten damage. One of hundreds. I live with Celiac Disease myself, almost died from it. In retrospect, I realize I lost family members to it, and I'm still saying forget Celiac, it's a small speck in the bigger picture. Stanford Medicine released a paper called "What the Gut Can Teach Us About Migraine"[80], but really, it's what the gut can teach us about our entire being.

The side effects of gluten create multi-tiered issues. We know dental decay is rampant with gluten sensitivity. What most don't know is that root canals feed depression. It's an indirect cause with significant consequences. The dark shadow ends up lurking constantly, so you need to continuously be countering its effects. *Unfortunately,* I know this one firsthand too.

"Dental health and "leaky teeth" may be intimately linked to the etiology and course of depression, while significantly impacting quality of life."[81]

The magnitude of damage gluten can do is surreal. Literally, surreal. I know it's a lot to take in. Hang in there, I'm giving you all the science and facts to eliminate any doubts, learn it once and you'll never need to read about gluten again...

Systemic Damage

"Systemic", in medical terms, means full body. Systemic gluten damage means:
1) Inside (brain, cells, organs, nerves, blood...)
2) Outside (skin, hair loss, physical stature, bones/teeth)
3) And the ethers (emotions, mood, mental capacity)

This book is focused on brain damage, but there's a key element about gluten you have to understand, which requires a systemic overview. That element is: For something knocking the lights out of your immune system, which is your only natural defense system, you become susceptible to all illness.

Triggering an autoimmune disease often launches The Domino Effect with your health. "People already affected by a first autoimmune disease have a higher probability of being affected by a second autoimmune disorder."[82] ...That's because their system is compromised and can't fight things off anymore.

When you understand that gluten creates chaos in your body, and that chaos can be expressed in every disorder that exists, you understand gluten. It's the same as asking "What can fire burn?" Answer: Everything, it can even melt steel if you give it time.

AUTOIMMUNE DESTRUCTION IS A PITFALL

Science is calling Celiac Disease the pitfall to hundreds of other diseases:

"Coeliac disease and autoimmune Addison's disease: a clinical pitfall"[83]

"High frequency of coeliac disease among patients with autoimmune adrenocortical failure"[84]

"Prospective screening for coeliac disease in patients with Graves' hyperthyroidism using anti-gliadin and tissue transglutaminase antibodies"[85]

"The prevalence of coeliac disease in adult diabetes mellitus"[86]

"[Chronic Hepatitis Due to Gluten Enteropathy] We would like to stress on the diverse clinical manifestations of celiac disease and the importance of serologic screening with antibodies to tissue transglutaminase in differential diagnosis of chronic liver disease"[87]

"Prevalence of gluten-sensitive celiac disease in women with reproductive dysfunction"[88]...

"Reproductive dysfunction" makes you think it's only infertility, when actually, spontaneous abortion is also an effect (two of the subjects in that very study miscarried). How many couples have lost their babies and never even knew why? Impossible to know. But is it acceptable for even one baby to die due to toxic food that their mother thought was the "staff of life" and their doctor told them they were safe to eat?

That last study is from Russia and it'll probably never see light of day in North America. Many of these studies, from the 1990's and even earlier, link Celiac and NCGS to some pretty serious issues and suggest screening early. Hundreds of studies, thousands of specific case studies, thousands of direct links, and decades later, we haven't progressed much. If anything, we're regressing because food companies are pushing back and sponsoring corrupt studies to muddy the waters even further. Confusion creates fear, and fear creates denial/non-action.

Millions of people are going through life thinking they have all these different disorders, and they will go to their grave never knowing they could have been healthy, had they just removed gluten from their life.

I can still feel the hug around me and tears rubbing from her face to mine... A woman who had miscarried for years, never got past first trimester, and was now at 8 1/2 months. She came to see me at a talk I did in Texas, to say it was a radio interview she heard me on that finally got her to go gluten free, regardless of test results. She had tested negative for Celiac twice and had been put on anti-depressants. What she and her husband went through is criminal. (last message I got, baby #1 was a girl and she was 7 months pregnant with baby #2)

NCGS CREATES SYSTEMIC DAMAGE AS MUCH AS CELIAC

"It is now accepted that **gluten sensitivity is a systemic illness** that can manifest in a range of organ systems... Such manifestations can occur independently of the presence of the classic small-bowel lesion that defines CD."[89]

Layman's Terms: NCGS can cause total body damage, while still showing zero damage on intestinal biopsy, ruling out Celiac. Remember when I said biopsy is useless?

DIAGNOSES AT AUTOPSY

In many cases, Celiac Disease is diagnosed at autopsy, not biopsy. I'm not being dramatic. Yes, I'm passionate about people losing their lives, but I never speak on this topic without facts. Celiac Disease is never the cause of death on an autopsy. And yet:

"CD was found to be associated with an 8-fold increased risk of death from liver cirrhosis... Hypertransaminasemia has been reported in about 40% of adults and in 54% of children with a classical presentation of CD at the time of diagnosis."[90]

If 40-54% of patients have liver disease at the time of Celiac diagnoses, and the medical data is telling us 8x premature death for those people, how many autopsies that name the cause of death as liver cirrhosis should actually say Celiac Disease? Their liver heals when they go gluten free, so why are we allowing this to continue?? All this chaos, for a replaceable loaf of bread. *Highly profitable bread.*

QUICK MENTION REGARDING DOCTORS

I've done my share of ranting about negligence, misdiagnoses, and condescending tones. I just want to go on the record and say I'm not bitter, nor am I bashing all doctors. Just like every profession on earth, there are good and bad ones (including my profession). It's a compliment that I hold them to a high standard. And perhaps I've had too many people cry on my shoulder because someone finally told them they're not crazy and don't need to be on pain killers or anti-depressants for the rest of their life.

"First, do no harm" is the only famous part of the Hippocratic Oath. Kind of vague. Here's a bit more from the oath: "I will use those dietary regimens which will benefit my patients according to my greatest ability and judgment, and I will do no harm or injustice to them. I will not give a lethal drug to anyone."[357]

Not give a lethal drug to anyone... a quarter of a million people a year die from prescribed drugs and suicides from anti-depressants. But don't worry, the system has things covered, less and less doctors are taking the oath anymore[358]. Do no harm, dietary regime, not giving lethal drugs are all outdated, so let's do away with the oath.

Scientists Call Gluten...

TOXIC, POISONS

"**Toxic** gliadin peptides"[91]

"...certain cereal products represent **poisons** that not only destroy small intestinal mucosa..."[92]

"The **toxic** protein fractions of gluten include gliadins and glutenins"[93]

THEY ALSO CALL IT AN EPIDEMIC

Astounding, isn't it? You can have a full-on epidemic in plain sight, have scientists actually call it an epidemic, right in the studies published in major journals, and still, it remains almost invisible and even mocked in the media more than anything else. Unfortunately, we have several health epidemics happening simultaneously, so it's easy to get lost in the shuffle.

"EPIDEMIC" CENTRAL AMERICA

These scientists are based in the Netherlands but did a wide study of Central American countries as wheat sweeps its way in, bringing European and North American wheat-related diseases with it.

Their objective is: "...to alert authorities responsible for the planning of education and health, to find possibilities to avoid a rise in these disorders before the epidemics start, as has occurred in the Mediterranean countries."[94]

"HIDDEN EPIDEMIC" EASTERN EUROPE

More than one study and group of scientists are using the word epidemic. The actual title of this study: "Recognising coeliac disease in Eastern Europe--the hidden epidemic in our midst?"[95]

"CD... GLOBAL VILLAGE"

As time goes on, we'll keep seeing scientists say:

"...celiac disease is the most common food intolerance in the world...

...there is a wide spectrum of its clinical presentation (classical, atypical, silent and latent forms of celiac disease) ...

...celiac disease is spread worldwide as in a common "Global Village", and greater levels of awareness and attention on gluten intolerance are needed, both in the Old and in the New World."[96]

"PUBLIC HEALTH PROBLEM"

This study calls CD "a new and challenging public health problem", note the fact that they know it affects everyone, not just those with CD:

"The availability of new, simple, very sensitive and specific serological tests (anti-gliadin, anti-endomysium and anti-transglutaminase antibody assays) have shown that celiac disease is common not only in Europe and in people of European ancestry but also in the developing countries where the major staple diet is wheat (Southern Asia, the Middle East, North West and East Africa, South America), ...

...**both in the general population** and in the groups at risk... ["groups at risk" is referring to CD and NCGS]

...Gluten intolerance thus appears to be a widespread public health problem and an increased level of awareness and clinical suspicion are needed in the New World where physicians must learn to recognize the variable clinical presentations (classical, atypical and silent forms) of celiac disease."[97]

You have one group calling for awareness using blood (serological) tests, but the authorities who define conditions, decide what goes into medical textbooks and medical schools, which is what MD's are bound by, are sticking to the flawed biopsy, only at stage 4, as the only way to be diagnosed and the only people they'll acknowledge as affected. It's negligent.

"MIDDLE EAST, INDIA, NORTH AFRICA"

"Following the application of simple serological tests for the diagnosis of coeliac disease (CD) in the 1980s, it gradually became clear that the prevalence of CD in different countries in the Middle East, North Africa and India is almost the same as that in Western countries."[98]

THE REPUBLIC OF GLUTEN FREE

An epidemic in every wheat-eating country, a global village of sufferers… as devastating as the reality is, the wonderful thing is that you don't need to wait until the entire world comes around to the facts. Here, now, as you read this, you can instantly be a citizen of The Republic of GlutenFree. No passport or visa required. No bureaucratic red tape. You can make an instant decision to keep yourself out of the epidemic and step on to safe soil. We welcome you to our tribe, anytime you're ready. I'll personally be there to greet you at the door with a refreshing healing drink.

Given everything you know so far, let's compare to what's online.

The paradox of advertising is that sensationalized awful things sell really well... as long as they're happening to someone else. The minute you start talking about a food the viewer is eating daily, you're repelling that viewer and they'll click away as fast as possible. That's a loss of advertising income. Loss of ad income = death of a site/magazine.

ARTICLE #1 DECONSTRUCTED

Posted by Insider,[99] which is big enough for people to assume credibility. But just for safe measure, add someone "registered" to the mix: "INSIDER turned to registered dietitian RH for a crash course on the basic substance."

1) MD's and gastroenterologists have been missing the mark for 100+ years, but a registered dietitian with zero formal gluten education is an expert (no disrespect to her, she thinks she's being helpful... though you'd never catch me being quoted on a serious medical topic I haven't exhaustively studied).

2) She's going to give a crash course in 1 minute, on a topic I need a 10-hour course to cover the basics with, and 3 full days if I go into full details. I'll give her the benefit of the doubt, I can certainly create fact-filled bullet points, though I wouldn't call it a crash course.

THE HEADLINE: "Everything you need to know about gluten – and why it isn't as bad as you think"
...Immediately promising good news and telling you that you can keep eating anything you want. Essentially saying: *We're telling you what you want to hear, so click here, make yourself feel better (even though you're taking an antacid as you read it), and hopefully you'll click on the ad selling shampoo so we can renew our contract with our sponsor.*

IMAGE ON THE ARTICLE: "Joey" from the hit show "Friends", eating a slice of pizza. ...Who would want to see an image of brain lesions and someone mistakenly put in a psyche ward, sedated, and medicated for 23 years? And who doesn't love Joey?? He's adorable, and now tied to pizza.

MISINFORMATION WILDFIRE: The term I've been using for bad information getting repeated so much, it spreads like wildfire everywhere. Actual quotes from the article:

"It affects less than 1%"

"While it is possible to simply be intolerant to gluten, those sensitivities are less widely understood and far less serious"
...Far less serious? Dementia, depression, arthritis, and twice the inflammation and morbidity rates as Celiac Disease is far less serious?

"A recent study by Harvard Medical School also indicated that an unnecessary gluten-free diet can cause heart problems."
...Everyone piggyback on the big Harvard name, and if you skipped that chapter, I cover this myth in the Gluten Myths section. You can see it's still getting traction a year later, all these bad articles do.

Great job on the crash course. Using the same amount of space, an informed person would have said:
-We're learning CD is a lot more common than 1%
-NCGS is 6x more prevalent and equally or more harmful
-It's important to replace gluten choices with healthy GF foods and not just anything labeled GF

Most people yapping about gluten are only reading Internet articles to learn about it, which keeps feeding Misinformation Wildfire. If this dietitian had taken my course or done as much research and reading on her own (studies, not Internet articles), she wouldn't be able to spew myths, not ethically anyways.

You're thinking: "A dietitian on an entertainment site can make errors, but surely if it's an MD on a medical site..." I hear you. Let's go to a renowned cardiologist on a medical site...

ARTICLE #2 DECONSTRUCTED

"With such a constellation of symptoms, it's not surprising that gluten is being blamed for a host of ailments, but the truth is that only people with celiac disease get sick from eating it."[100]

?!?!?!!?!?!?!!?

The first time I saw that quote, I thought it was a hoax. I pray he's better at heart surgery than his knowledge of gluten. The good doc goes on in that same article: "There are people who need to stay away from gluten, but, for most of us, paying more for gluten-free foods, or going out of our way to buy them, is just another food scam."

If your doctor sounds anything like the one on this page, get a new doctor. I'm not saying that to be fresh, I'm saying it for your safety. They're not gods, they don't know everything. If you suspect gluten issues, then you need to find a doctor who can help you instead of comparing grocery bills and sharing kitten videos on Facebook with you.

We used to have to worry about doctors and "God Complex". Now we need to add "Celebrity Complex" to the list and squeeze ourselves into their schedule between radio interviews, TV appearances, online summits, conferences, blogs, tweets, podcasts, and book tours (When do they have time to read and stay on top of the newest science?)

REPETITION CREATES A PERCEPTION OF REALITY

When the average person sees this stuff hundreds of times with "Harvard" and "registered dietitian" or "MD" ... well, *you know what happens.*

When you see information on gluten, ask: Is the person providing the information working exclusively within the world of gluten and Celiac Disease? Have they read thousands of pages of data and studies, or are they just parrots re-tweeting and re-killing people with what they saw on the Internet themselves.

Moral of the Story: Ignore everything you read on the Internet about gluten, NCGS, and Celiac Disease. If you had a brain tumor, you'd go to a neurologist, not the Internet. Gluten damage is just as serious and can be a cause of that very tumor and other cancers.[101] Don't take it less seriously just because it's food related. Assume that nothing on the Internet will be accurate about gluten for another 33 years, probably longer.

HOW ARE YOU DOING?

Take a break for a minute, I've thrown a lot at you here. Maybe use that minute to go online and write a review of this book, even though we're only halfway through, because you can only imagine how much more I have for you. You will literally be saving the life of someone who reads your review and gets this book as a result of it. I thank you in advance, *and they thank you in advance.*

The only solution I see to the whole problem is word of mouth. I just can't see the medical system acting for several more decades. The legal system is wound up by corporate ponor$hip. I'm counting on you to share, so are your co-humans who have no idea about all this.

BRAIN DAMAGE

Obviously, more than gluten is causing brain damage. There's no way to cover every toxin on earth and that's not what this book is about, but I'll cover a few food-related brain toxins that are most commonly crossing your path, many of which are being marketed to you as health food. Caveat Emptor *(buyer beware).* You can't avoid poison if you don't know how to recognize it. Their job is to sell, your job is to know better. First, more regarding Your Brain on Gluten...

Brain Damage Spectrum

If I said headaches were the same thing as dementia, just on a smaller scale, you'd probably think I was eating gluten again and my brain was fried. But the medical system does this every day...

AUTISM is still autism whether we're talking about:
1) A piano-playing genius who has some difficulty socializing
2) Mute, unresponsive, violent, needs restraints and sedation

DEPRESSION is still depression whether we're talking about:
1) Suicidal, in the E.R./psyche ward for cutting wrists
2) Mood swings, sad for no reason, but works/functions

Newer studies are looking at brain disorders together and not separating them anymore, with gut damage standing out as one of the most common causes: "Gut microbiota in autism and mood disorders." [102]

BRAIN AND MOOD SPECTRUMS

No one goes from being deliriously happy on Monday to suicidal on Tuesday. There's a time lapse between those two things. So why would headaches during 20's, turning into dementia decades later, be a big stretch? If anything, it's the logical progression. They're on opposite ends of the same neurological spectrum.

Everything around you is a spectrum. Your thoughts, feelings, marriage (you don't go from being in love on Saturday to divorce on Sunday). Everything both tangible and intangible are on a slide ruler. Your health is the same.

Headache / depression / brain fog are on one end of the spectrum. Dementia / schizophrenia / bi-polar are on the other. In between those things are a long list of neurological disorders, some you've never heard of (what on earth is tardive dyskinesia), others you've accepted as a normal part of your life (headaches).

Do you consider 34 BILLION dollars in over-the-counter medication normal? We went from $16B (still insane) to $34B in less than a decade.[103] That's just the United States. Care to know where the U.S. is with prescription medication as I write this? $811,000,000,000. That's 811 billion, projected to grow to $1,060,000,000,000 within 3 years.

That number is growing because people are sliding down the same spectrum you're on right now, with Alzheimer's leading the way. Depression, of course, always continues to grow. What do you suppose the advertising budgets are for 811 billion-dollar sales?

THE DEEP END, AND WHY IT SHOULD MATTER TO YOU

I often avoid using the word schizophrenia because it's "so far out there" that people tune out. The problem is, it's *not* far out there. Schizophrenia is like every other neurological issue: It starts small and grows. Dementia will be a diagnosable disease for over half our population in this lifetime. How far out there does that sound to you? Over 50% of everyone around you will have neurological disease by 2033, many of them severe and debilitating forms of dementia. The future is here, which is why this book isn't messing around or sugar coating.

The reason perfectly healthy people should be paying attention: No one goes from normal to psyche ward overnight. It's important to know the full scale and how someone gets from one end to the other (how can you avoid drowning in the deep end of the pool if you don't know where it is?)

Please keep reading. My goal isn't to scare or throw useless stats at you (we both have much better things to do). The goal is to put such strong knowledge in your mind, that you'll become immune to the fluff and silly noise on the Internet and you'll know all the factors that cause mental decline and what to do about it *today*. You trusted me and bought this book, keep trusting me through the next few challenging chapters.

WHY I'M HIGHLIGHTING SCHIZOPHRENIA...

...Because if schizophrenia can disappear with one diet change, imagine how much easier it is to be rid of depression. To be clear, I'm not undermining how painful depression is. It's a dark, lonely, painful place and the number one cause of disability in the world, tormenting over 300 million people, causing 800,000 suicides a year worldwide.[104]

Believe me, I'm not making light of it, and as someone who fell into clinical depression myself, I would never make light of it. It was horrific to be in that dark tunnel and feel like there was no way out. I remember once thinking "What if this is my new existence?

What if I'll never be well again? How will I work and support myself?" It was terrifying.

Depression can put such dark sunglasses on your eyes, you forget a sun even exists, and I've been there. But compared to wild hallucinations and stabbing someone 99 times because spiders are eating them...

"Schizophrenia is frequently found in people with Celiac Disease and Celiac Disease is frequently found in people with schizophrenia ... In cultures where gluten grains are rarely eaten, schizophrenia is rare or non-existent."[105]

Remember the 1% myth, and the fact that 40% are susceptible with the genes, most are undiagnosed, and NCGS is 6x more prevalent and causing the same brain damage. We know schizophrenia is common with gluten damage, so what's the math? How many are susceptible? *Right.* I'll keep going...

When Western grains were introduced to the South Pacific Islands, schizophrenia went up to 1 in 100, from 1 in 30,000[106] !!!!!!!! (I needed a deep yoga breath, *and drink,* when I saw that)

Grains took a population of over 2 million people, who made no other food change other than introducing grains, and turned that number to one in a hundred almost overnight. 1 in 100 means if you walked in any downtown city, you'd encounter a schizophrenic person every few seconds. That's a big difference from 1 in 30,000.

WWII: Wheat shortages showed us a decrease in hospitalization rates for schizophrenic patients. When the war was over, wheat became available again and hospitalization rates went right back up.[107] Same patients, schizophrenic on grains, normal off grains, no other changes.

As early as 1953, Bender noted that "children with schizophrenia were prone to having celiac disease."[108] Over 6 decades later, if you say gluten and schizophrenia, everyone screams "witch" and says you're blowing things out of proportion. The truth is just too much for most people to accept, and I get why. It doesn't change the facts. What I tell people is: "Face the truth while you still have the mental capacity to do so and can take counter-measures."

OUR INSTINCTS FAIL US WHEN SOMETHING IS SCARY

My books (and I) got crucified in reviews in 2009 because I wrote about several studies showing oats doing damage to Celiacs. 8 years later, Health Canada declares oats are doing too much damage to the gut to be classified as gluten free anymore, and now oats are officially not seen as gluten free by the Government of Canada (though the grocery shelves are still filled with "Certified GF Oats", which is where my "controversial" A to Z Safe/Unsafe list would help you). I'll deal with the bad reviews if it saves some lives.

It takes time for us to accept things sometimes. Gluten and schizophrenia is one of those things. It's just too scary a place to go. The working title of this very book was originally "Gluten Psychosis" (would you still have bought it?), and then I changed it last minute.

As you keep reading, suspend your fears, and suspend the instinctive reaction of thinking "No, that's too serious, it can't just be gluten, those people must have something else going on."

But they usually don't. I didn't. There are thousands of case studies of people with dementia, schizophrenia, bi-polar... people who have been medicated and often even spent years locked up in psychiatric wards, who became normal within weeks or months of removing gluten from their diet, were released, and continued to live symptom-free productive lives.

SCHIZOPHRENIA CASE STUDY[109] 29-year-old woman, diagnosed with "autistic disorder, social / occupational dysfunction, affective flattening, and inferential thinking". They ignored her diarrhea and weight loss at first, focused on her behavioral problems. She could have been diagnosed correctly from the start, she had classic gastro symptoms, which should have made it easier.

Age 33: "The diagnosis of schizophrenia was made. She was treated with Fluphenazine, Thioridazine and Lorazepam."

Age 35: "Psychiatric symptoms of affective flattening, avolition (lack of desire, motivation, or persistence), autistic behaviour, auditory hallucinations, telepathic thought and catastrophic expectations were still present...diagnosis of schizophrenia was again confirmed..."

EEG showed brain was "normal". Like mine did when I was debilitated and losing feeling on my left side.

Finally, they stopped ignoring her weight loss and malnutrition issue and "...Celiac Disease was diagnosed and treated with Gluten Free Diet **with quick improvement in a few days.** After 6 months the patient's body weight reached 50 kg [her normal weight], **blood chemistry and histology all returned to normal...**"

A year later, she was still completely free of symptoms, off all medication, zero neuro issues, living a normal healthy life.

The doctors suggest in their conclusion that schizophrenia might be more of a symptom than a disease: "...After a follow-up of 1 year the patient is still asymptomatic... Schizophrenic symptoms may be the expression of organic disease, such as CD, rather than primary psychiatric illness."

How many years of her life did this woman lose? You can be sure she didn't go from perfect at age 28 to psychiatric ward at age 29. She lost all her 20's, 30's, perhaps even childhood and teens. Maybe never got married and had kids. Medicated, didn't pursue career or business. ...whatever her dreams were, gone. She lost decades. *For gluten.* For god damn gluten. Sorry, I'm doing my best to watch my language, but I could have easily been her, so can you, so can your child, neighbor, sister, brother, spouse, ...

It's not just schizophrenia that has disappeared in thousands of cases with no change other than removing gluten from the person's diet, it's Alzheimer's[110], Parkinson's[111], MS,[112] ADHD,[113] Brain Fog[114], and all neurological issues on the spectrum of brain disorders. Regarding brain fog, that last study also remarks that the symptoms go away in both Celiac and Crohn's after 12 months GF.

CROHN'S SIDE NOTE: Because raw foods are not possible before healing, many Crohn's sufferers end up relying more heavily on grains. That may keep them perpetually sick. SOLUTION: Eliminate all grains and use quinoa (pseudo-grain), chia (seed), lentil, chick pea in savory foods, any nut or coconut flours in sweet foods/desserts. Use the safe GF flour list in the last section of this book. By the way, people keep arguing what quinoa is classified as (grain or pseudo), here's my answer: It's classified as no study is showing a single person reacting and it doesn't have lectins & co.

"DEMENTIA FROM GLUTEN-CONTAINING GRAINS"

They'll eventually identify various gluten-induced forms of dementia. The Mayo Clinic is calling deceased dementia patients found with gluten antibodies in their cortex "gluten encephalopathy: dementia from gluten-containing grains."[115] Hopefully we'll eventually do better than catching it only during autopsy. Hopefully, some of you reading this will help a friend or family member or patient get off gluten and see reversal or improvement of their condition. I can't wait to see those success stories.

TANGIBLE AND INTANGIBLE DAMAGE

Although we can measure gluten damage several ways: Intestinal biopsy, antibodies in blood, brain lesions on MRI... note that the outer effects include both intangible (depression) and tangible (epilepsy and bilateral brain calcification[116]) damage.

I'm not suggesting every neurological issue in the world is caused by gluten (though I might be naïve in saying that, when, exactly, did depression hit humanity? Was it 10,000 years ago?) We can safely say gluten isn't strengthening anybody by guaranteeing holes in their gut.

The cause *is* gluten a whole lot more often than your mind can process right now. I've read the thousands of case studies, I feel like I know these people personally and I feel devastated at the years they've lost. Sometimes, their entire lives. We can stop this. You and I can stop this. This book is the snowball, waiting for you to push it down the mountain and grow so it creates awareness. Awareness + action = change. We can finally use the share button to help instead of misinform.

"An association between many psychiatric and gluten-related disorders has been known for some time."[117]

Gluten and Depression

"**Depression** is reported to be a feature of coeliac disease and is ranked as **its most common neuropsychiatric disturbance.**"[118]

The reason gluten and depression often come together (besides actual chemicals shooting into your bloodstream and brain) is that gluten, overall, creates chaos in your system. It's a systemic [total body] problem that brings your body down. Depression, by definition, is going down... *depressing.* It's a verb, it's not a noun. You don't "get" depression the way you get a virus. Depression is something you "do" (involuntarily).

Depression is practically a given with Celiac Disease. As the numbers start piling up with more studies on Gluten Sensitivity, headaches seem to accompany NCGS as much as they do CD. Myself included, I've met very few people with gluten issues who didn't have a long history of headaches both mild and severe, which is exactly what the data shows...

"...high frequency of headaches in patients with CD and vice versa with a beneficial effect of a gluten-free diet. Screening for CD could be advised in the diagnostic work-up of patients with headache."[119]

"Children with untreated coeliac disease are characteristically unhappy and after a few days of treatment with a gluten-free diet their mood improves. This improvement in mood can be rapidly reversed by introducing gluten into their diet again."[120]

SEROTONIN / TRYPTOPHAN DEPLETION

The Department of Psychiatry, University of Pittsburgh School of Medicine, fed rats 5 proteins: Zein (corn/maize), wheat gluten, soy protein isolate, casein, lactalbumin. Zein caused the biggest drop in serotonin, followed by wheat gluten and casein.[121] *R.I.P., rats were killed in that study while their brains and blood were examined.*

The results weren't different in a human study[122] measuring tryptophan after consuming zein, wheat gluten, α-Lactalbumin (protein/dairy). Since tryptophan affects serotonin, as well as other things, this matters. *No humans were sacrificed in this study, other than the gluten/dairy damage, maybe even saved them via awareness.*

Connect the dots: We know gluten (including corn/maize gluten) and dairy decrease tryptophan, and "Children with autism have a higher deficiency of tryptophan than the control group of healthy children. Lower levels of tryptophan may lead to the worsening of autistic symptoms such as mild depression and increased irritability."[123]

These children are reacting to several things in several ways, the accumulation of hits to their system is often too much. Removing one assault might lessen the symptoms, sometimes even seem like full recovery, but without testing all possible antibodies, how would you be sure there isn't underlying damage happening that will manifest years later? If that was my child, you can be sure I'd remove all known assaults: Gluten, grains, corn, dairy, and sugar. What's left to eat? Pure foods, exactly what we should all be eating.

DIGESTIVE DISORDERS AND DEPRESSION

It's always interesting when studies not originally looking at Celiac or NCGS find their way to it. The gut-brain connection is undeniable, and gluten damages both. In this case, a group of psychiatrists looking for the connection between digestive disorders and depression, and what is the number one disorder to hit their radar? They even mention the spectrum:

"One of the mostly recognized examples is coeliac disease where patients endure the large spectrum of psychopathological symptoms, starting with attention deficit all the way down to the intellectual disability... The dominant mental disease mentioned in this article is depression."[124] That was Poland.

This is Hungary, again, not looking at CD specifically, they were studying "Neurological and psychiatric aspects of some gastrointestinal diseases", and what disorder do they find themselves with: "Up to 85% of patients with histologically proven coeliac disease have no gastrointestinal symptoms; consequently, measurement of antigliadin antibody titre is therefore vital in all cases of idiopathic ataxia. Complete resolution of neurological symptoms is the result of gluten-free diet."[125]

Again and again and again:
1) No gastrointestinal symptoms
2) Antibodies in their blood
3) Neurological symptoms resolved by going gluten-free

"Celiac disease can manifest as psychiatric disorders like depression, anxiety or psychosis. Coincidence with eating disorders was also described. Usually proper diagnosis is performed secondary to psychiatric symptoms. In some cases gluten-free diet can reduce or even resolve both gastrointestinal and psychiatric symptoms."[126]

"Usually proper diagnosis is performed secondary to psychiatric symptoms" means you're usually diagnosed with a mental disorder first and treated with drugs. CD is never considered or screened until the patient stays sick or worsens, and no drug in the world is helping because they are continuing to eat the foods that are making their brain ill.

Antibodies and Brain Inflammation

"In 2010, an estimated 35.6 million people worldwide were living with dementia, a number that is expected to double in 20 years."[127]

I'm sorry this is so science heavy. I want to be sure it doesn't sound like me speaking and you're seeing unbiased, purely scientific evidence. I've made it easier by summarizing without medical jargon in the headlines, and some simplified explanations after study quotes.

INCREASED GLIADIN ANTIBODIES WITH BI-POLAR

"Individuals with bipolar disorder have increased levels of IgG antibodies to gliadin."[128] That means antibodies to gluten, but not necessarily intestinal damage and they would test negative for Celiac for their entire lifetime and be told they should eat "healthy whole grains" every day.

PSYCHOSIS, SCHIZOPHRENIA, ANTIBODIES=YES, CELIAC=NO (this affects 100% of the population)

"Individuals with recent-onset psychosis and with multi-episode schizophrenia who have increased antibodies to gliadin may share some immunologic features of celiac disease, **but their immune response to gliadin differs from that of celiac disease.**"[129]

SCHIZOPHRENIA WITH GLUTEN ANTIBODIES, NO GENES FOR CELIAC

"These findings indicate that the anti-gliadin immune response in schizophrenia has a different antigenic specificity from that in celiac disease and is independent of the action of transglutaminase enzyme and HLA-DQ2/DQ8. Meanwhile, the presence of elevated levels of antibodies to specific gluten proteins points to shared immunologic abnormalities in a subset of schizophrenia patients."[130]

ANTIBODIES CROSS BLOOD/BRAIN BARRIER AND CREATE BRAIN INFLAMMATION

"...a high correlation of IgG-mediated antibodies between the periphery and cerebral spinal fluid in schizophrenia but not healthy controls, particularly AGA IgG suggesting that these antibodies may be crossing the blood-brain barrier with resulting neuroinflammation."[131]

Imagine the level of toxin we're talking about for those antibodies to make their way into your spinal fluid. It goes right up your spine and shoots into your brain like a fire hose. That glutened brain has no chance, it's a sitting duck waiting to be shot.

"Patients with CD were more prone to develop neurologic disorders (51.4%) in comparison with control subjects (19.9%). These disorders include hypotonia, developmental delay, learning disorders and ADHD, headache, and cerebellar ataxia...

...the variability of neurologic disorders that occur in CD is broader than previously reported and includes "softer" and more common neurologic disorders, such as chronic headache, developmental delay, hypotonia, and learning disorders or ADHD."[132]

Hypotonia is "floppy baby syndrome", technically muscle atrophy. Who would ever connect gluten to that? Question for discussion: Some muscle atrophy, but still walks and functions normally, can be seen as a minor problem. What if that kid has dreams of being an athlete and can't so much as make tryouts? It'll casually get swept under the rug as "She was just born that way, not very athletic, clumsy kid." *What if that was Steffi Graf?*

Children on the Spectrum

Want to get me angry? I mean, throw-a-vase-across-the-room and have people ducking for cover angry? Tell me that a 5-year-old is about to be put on drugs. But it's not one child, it's millions of children. Get a counter out so you can record how many WTF moments you have in the next few minutes...

SOBERING NUMBERS

1997-2000: Anti-psychotic drugs increased by 138%, anti-depressants 42%, SSRIs 18%

1993-2000: Global use of these medications rose 300%

Combinations of drugs given to children, meaning two or more drugs given simultaneously, *to children,* increased 500%.

1997: Congress changed the law to allow drug ads to not be required to list all side effects (like violence and suicide). With the help of Madison Avenue and "condition branding" (you didn't think MadMen was fictional, did you?) ...The next 10 years saw a 700% increase in drug sales (combined, child and adult drugs), and it continues to grow year after year, as do SSRI induced suicides in children and adults.

We know these drugs cause violence and suicide, but instead of banning them, we fund research centers to figure what combination of drugs will cause the lesser number of suicides.[133] *(I'll refrain from saying what's on the tip of my tongue right now and just stick to the facts)*
Not only do we measure which medley might cause the lesser number of fatalities, we also measure which drugs and combinations cause violent methods of suicide versus non-violent suicide.[134] The UK did a study sampling all suicides committed in Sweden 1992-2004. Out of 1958 suicides with traces of SSRI's in their system during autopsy, 63.7% used violent means to end their lives.[135] We're analyzing these stats, but never questioning the use of these drugs. *(This time, I'm not refraining, I just have no words)*

...If you're wondering what this has to do with gluten, there's a high probability a gluten sufferer will be strongly encouraged to take anti-depressants, by multiple doctors, before and after diagnoses. You should know what you're getting into.

1 IN 6 CHILDREN

"1 in 6 children in the United States had a developmental disability in 2006-2008, ranging from mild disabilities such as speech and language impairments to serious developmental disabilities, such as intellectual disabilities, cerebral palsy, and autism."[136]

...must be some quack making up those crazy numbers...

That's a direct quote from the CDC (Centers for Disease Control and Prevention) of the United States of America. That's a government issued, medically documented number. 1 in 6 children with brain damage of some kind (that we know of, it's not like the impoverished and people with no insurance are taking their children to doctors, and their diets are usually the worst, making those numbers even more staggering).

Anti-depressants are creating disorders that never even existed before. "Serotonin Syndrome"[137]?!?

ADHD

"All ADHD-like symptomatology patients should be tested for CD with serum screening tests, as CD could be one of the causes of these neuropsychiatric symptoms. We are convinced that untreated CD may predispose to important mental and behavioral disorders."[138]

...The important element to that study was that after 6 months gluten-free, every single kid improved. That's why they suggest immediately screening for CD when a kid has ADHD symptoms.

"ADHD-like symptomatology is markedly overrepresented among untreated CD patients and that a gluten-free diet may improve symptoms significantly within a short period of time."[139]

OBSESSIVE COMPULSIVE DISORDER

Remember the spectrum factor... a 7-year-old diagnosed with OCD[140] will probably display what at age 27? 57? 67? If the OCD is severe or affects normal life functions, the child will most likely be pegged autistic. Then what? What's the Gluten Path for these children? This question keeps me awake at night and haunts me through the day.

By the way, the 7-year-old was an actual case study and after 60 days gluten-free: "OCD symptoms had improved 80% and his anxiety had improved 90% since the last visit... His eczema was 100% improved. The patient ate only gluten-free food and used gluten-free personal care products."

6 months later, the mother "reported 1 instance of a relapse in symptoms of irritation and anxiety the day after the child had eaten food that had been cross-contaminated with food containing gluten from another family member."

AUTISM

Gluten Antibodies found in: 87% autistic children versus 1% normal kids[141]

It's important to note we're talking about antibodies, not necessarily stage 4 "total villous atrophy" *(yet)*.

Besides the avoidable harm to the child, the other problem is that if we wait for official Celiac Disease diagnosis, we're misleading the population into thinking that the link between autism and gluten aren't common enough to cause alarm.

This is Key: If (stage 4) Celiac and Autism are linked at 5%, it doesn't ring 5-alarm bells. What about 87% of autistic kids with gluten antibodies? What about 100% with harmful bacteria in their gut, does that warrant a fire bell? ...Yes, and it would affect Grain ale, so let's keep a lid on it.

Not only are we almost guaranteeing neurological damage to these children, but we're risking several other issues that are common with Celiac Disease, such as osteopenia [irreversible bone condition that causes decreased calcification, decreased density, or reduced mass].

Tunisia: "Most of the screened children showed an atypical and asymptomatic form, but even the typical forms were underdiagnosed. Osteopenia was frequently observed in celiac disease patients."[142]

Note that most of those children were asymptomatic. That's the deadly part of all this... no symptoms, and then 10-20-40 years later, they can have bone issues ranging from chronic back pain and herniated discs, to outright deformity. ...And no one will ever make the connection to gluten. I'd need 5000 more pages to this book if I covered every way gluten can damage the body, and the kind of long-term risks we have documented over the decades.

Also note that it's a worldwide problem. It's not a coincidence that I'm quoting studies from all over the world. I have dozens of other studies from Canada[143], United States[144], Finland[145], ... all showing abnormally low bone density or outright osteoporosis in people with Celiac. I chose Tunisia so that I cover the globe by the time I get to the end of this book.

It's not just Celiac and lower bone density, it's also NCGS, as a Russian study[146] showed. ALL issues you're seeing with Celiac, are also issues with NCGS. At some point, after I'm long dead, they'll acknowledge there's no difference with any of this, and that gluten is bad for the entire planet. Dr. Ford (New Zealand) said it decades ago.

Luckily, some doctors are catching it. A small boy with ongoing fractures was finally diagnosed with Celiac Disease (he had no other typical symptoms, just kept breaking bones). Once he was gluten-free, he suffered no further "recurrent bone fractures."[147] His asymptomatic brother was also diagnosed, preventing goodness only knows what issues in the long term.

I know I'm veering off the main focus of brain sometimes, but how can I have all this data and not provide some warnings? It would be morally wrong. A lot of these issues are symptoms that can help with earlier diagnosis.

DEPRESSION IN CHILDREN WITH CELIAC

We always think of depression as an adult problem. Children, especially those born in an unhealthy state, would never know the difference and never complain. I have a theory (which I pray will be wrong) that in another generation or two, no one will complain about depression because no one will know the difference. We've already tipped the scale further to the dark side, so why would that be a stretch? There are more medicated than non-medicated people in the developed world right now. My theory is already more than 50% reality.

CELIAC KIDS AT 40% HIGHER RISK OF SUICIDE

Completely unacceptable! 40% higher risk of suicide in teenagers with Celiac Disease.[148] Not just depression, *suicide.*

SCHIZOPHRENIA IN CHILDREN WITH CD

Brain disorders are generally neuro-degenerative and take time, but not exclusively. Just like I went from Iron Woman to I.V. in months, some people free-fall as quickly with neuro-degeneration. This isn't novel. The connection was made with Celiac children and schizophrenia in the 1950's.[149]

ALIEN BACTERIA

There have been many Moments of Truth on this journey, one of them being that scientists have found 35 sequences of "alien bacteria" (their term, not mine) in 20-40% of children with celiac disease.[150] Alien meaning they don't know what it is, can't scientifically identify any element of the bacteria. What's more, the bacteria are alive, they're reproducing themselves in the lab once extracted from these children's guts. What kind of disruption are those kids experiencing and what are they susceptible to? There's no way to answer that question because we have no idea what these alien living bacteria are.

When the gut is in chaos and invaded by aliens, while the bloodstream is flooded with harmful antibodies, how is a small child supposed to fight back? How is anyone, at any age, supposed to fight back? How long can that body and brain hold up the fight?

DEFINITION: pan·dem·ic
adjective
1. (of a disease) prevalent over a whole country or the world

TURKEY, AT LEAST ONE PSYCHIATRIC DISORDER IN 50% OF THE CELIAC KIDS

"Pediatric Quality of Life Inventory were significantly lower in children with celiac disease when compared to the control group (p<0.05). There was at least one psychiatric disorder in the 26 (50%) children with celiac disease..."[151]

SWEDEN, GREATER RISK OF PSYCHIATRIC DISORDERS

10,903 Swedish children with CD and 12,710 of their siblings: "...children with celiac disease had a 1.4-fold greater risk of future psychiatric disorders. Childhood celiac disease was identified as a risk factor for mood disorders, anxiety disorders, eating disorders, behavioral disorders, ADHD, ASD, and intellectual disability."[152]

SCANDINAVIA, CD LINKED TO UNDER-ACHIEVEMENT

They followed 2427 kids for 21 years. All from the same place, same economic status, same environmental factors, same schools, same everything... except for the children who were screened and diagnosed with Celiac Disease. 21 years later, here's the state of affairs:

"-Fewer Celiac subjects had a university or college degree (5.3% vs. 22.8%)

-Fewer Celiac subjects worked in managerial or professional positions (28% vs. 45%)

-Employment rate, as well as occupational classification and socioeconomic status suggested a **uniform tendency to underachievement by the Celiac subjects**...

-In children and adolescents with Celiac, we found a significant **increase in disruptive behavioral and depressive disorders.**"[153]

SAUDI ARABIA 2x THE NUMBERS

"Our study provided evidence of a high prevalence of CD among Saudi children... a rate that is at least twice the average prevalence rate in Europe and North America."[154]

DOWN SYNDROME AND CELIAC, CHINA

Minzu University of China analyzed 31 studies based on 4383 individuals: "These results demonstrated that patients (children) with Down syndrome had high prevalence of CD (more than one in twenty). The prevalence is high enough to motivate screening CD in DS children."[155]

DOWN SYNDROME AND CELIAC, INDIA

"The present results showed a high prevalence of CD in DS children in a tertiary hospital in India and low hemoglobin to be an important risk factor. The authors recommend that all Indian children with Down syndrome, particularly those with anemia should be screened for celiac disease."[156]

Celiac Disease has become a pandemic in both children and adults in the northern parts of India, where they eat more wheat than in other areas. Their government has set up a task force[157] to control the potential health crisis.

DOWN SYNDROME AND CELIAC, PORTUGAL

"DS Portuguese patients have a high CD prevalence rate. This study supports that, in our population, the current recommendations for CD screening in DS patients should be implemented and screening must be EMA based."[158]

DOWN SYNDROME AND CELIAC, BRAZIL

"These data indicates a high prevalence (5.6%) of confirmed celiac disease in Down syndrome patients from southern Brazil."[159]

5% IS REALLY HOW MANY? AND REMEMBER THE 1% MYTH

We have the same problem here as we do with Autism, the numbers aren't being communicated properly. All these studies are counting only stage 4, officially diagnosed, and we already know only 1 out of 9 are diagnosed. Plus, we need to add the 0-3 stages, as well as NCGS cases. What's the real number? No one knows because they're not usually testing for or recording any antibodies. It's a safe bet the number is *not* 5%. If 50-70% of Down's kids had CD or gluten antibodies, would it get your attention?

DECADES OF UNHEEDED WARNINGS

Pediatricians all over the world have been documenting gluten damage to children for decades *(I wonder what goes through their minds every time they hear the word fad)*.

New Zealand, Dr. Rodney Ford, pediatrician, gastroenterologist, allergy specialist, has been calling for a "gluten free planet" for 30+ years now. This isn't an MD who picks up a false Internet article between book tours, he's neck-deep in practice, has seen thousands of patients, knows the topic scientifically as well as first-hand case studies, has seen miraculous recoveries from GFD.

I interviewed him years ago, his frustration at the level of denial was audible. He deserves tremendous credit for not wavering when gluten was nowhere on the grand stage as it's starting to be now. He's a maverick and a champion. Total hall of famer.

French pediatrician Lachaux presented "Les formes cliniques trompeuses de la maladie cœliaque"[160] (translation: Misleading presentations of celiac).

I don't think it ever got translated or shown anywhere in the world. Children are being led down the wrong roads, misdiagnosed, medicated, their entire lives are being stolen from them. This paper wasn't from an obscure source, it was from the Unit of Hepatology, Gastroenterology and Pediatric Nutrition, Department of Pediatrics, Édouard-Herriot Hospital, Lyon, France.

BEYOND THE CONCLUSIONS

Sometimes the very titles and/or conclusions of studies are enough to create alarm. Three times higher risk of death in children with Celiac is alarming enough, but when you read beyond the conclusions, you really get full impact. Do you know what some of the reasons for that threefold increase in death are?

"All-cause mortality more than 5 yr after diagnosis was increased threefold in children... This excess mortality in children was primarily because of an increased risk of death from accidents, suicide, and violence... cancer... and cerebrovascular disease"[161]

Suicide and violence. Cerebrovascular Disease is abnormalities of blood vessels to the brain, cutting off oxygen and nutrients to the brain. From food. *Food.* Perhaps it's time to stop referring to gluten as food.

1969 we landed on the moon and the paper titled "Active coeliac disease in childhood"[162] was ignored. Are we too distracted by moon landings and Super Bowls to notice?

As a collective society, we're turning our eyes away from a train wreck that we can stop. There are too few people understanding the gravity of the situation.

"All wheat attack is not celiac"[163]
World Journal of Gastroenterology

BRAIN DAMAGE IS SLOW, DEGENERATIVE

It never happens overnight. I said it before, I'll say it again: No one is deliriously happy on Monday and suicidal on Tuesday. No one. Ever. Not anyone. Not anywhere. Not once. It's universal. Same for Alzheimer's: No one is ultra-sharp on Monday and can't identify their children on Tuesday, not unless we're talking blunt force trauma.

THE MAJORITY ARE ASYMPTOMATIC, REFERRED TO AS SILENT[164]

That's a really important key to all this: Most people are asymptomatic,[165] they show no symptoms at surface level. They don't show symptoms of any kind. Not gastrointestinal. Not neurological. Not anything that the average medical professional would recognize. But the damage is being done. If we looked for antibodies in their system, we'd immediately see issues. Those issues grow and eventually surface.

The fact that most people are asymptomatic means we need to be **proactive** and not **reactive**, and that's not a philosophy our society has embraced yet. "If it ain't broke, don't fix it" spells trouble for a lot of people.

WE CAN SEE / MEASURE GLUTEN INFILTRATE THE BRAIN

1) BLOOD TESTS
The least expensive and least invasive is to look for antibodies in the blood. If your doctor's a champ, they'll take it a step further and look for IEL's on top of antibodies. By identifying biomarkers, you're catching the smoke before there's a fire.

2) MRI (Magnetic Resonance Imaging)
Glutened brains will show brain lesions.[166] This is a decreased supply of blood to the brain (important?), called hypoperfusion, caused by inflammation. Decreased supply of blood to the brain for an extended period of time will lead to brain degeneration.

Cause and Cure: "All patients with both migraine and CD showed evident abnormalities in regional cerebral blood flow...the gluten free diet strongly affected the abnormalities."[167]

3) FOLLOW THE NEON LIGHT

There's yet another way to measure how gluten gets from gut to brain, and this study goes all the way back to 1978. They fed rats radioactively labeled gluten protein and it showed up in their brain as exorphins.[168]

Exorphins are molecules that aren't supposed to get to your brain, but with gluten, they get there.[169] There's a chemical addiction the brain and certain harmful gut microbes have to gluten that can make cravings the same as that for morphine and heroin. It all ends up as exorphins, which means your brain can't even tell the difference between morphine and gluten.

"Gluten can be degraded into several morphine-like substances, named gluten exorphins. These compounds have proven opioid effects and could mask the deleterious effects of gluten protein on gastrointestinal lining and function."[170]

4) SPECT (Single Photon Emission Computed Tomography)

"There's actually a SPECT study that people who are sensitive to gluten have lower blood flow to their brain when they're exposed to it."[171]

DAMAGE WITHOUT CROSSING BLOOD-BRAIN BARRIER, *IN EVERYONE*

Gluten is a complicated protein. We've only just begun breaking all its components down and studying their effects. Gluten exorphin B5 [GE-B5, from wheat] is just one of those components, and it "can modify brain neurotransmitter release without crossing the Blood-Brain Barrier."[172]

Note that is all brains, not just CD or NCGS, and we knew this over a decade ago. It doesn't stop there. GE-B5 has been proven to stimulate prolactin secretion[173] ...and this is where critical info for 100% of the population never leaves the science lab because who the heck knows what prolactin secretion is and who cares. Well, it's something that affects your pituitary gland, otherwise known as your brain's "master gland". Also called the "master of the endocrines."[174]

I, for one, am interested when a food protein starts playing darts on the master gland of my brain, and it's a bull's eye every time. This dart never misses.

CELL DAMAGE, NOT ALWAYS REVERSIBLE

"...advanced cell loss and, at some point of disease progression, deficits become irreversible."[175]

BRAIN SEIZURES, NOT ALWAYS REVERSIBLE

Trieste, Italy, Divisione di Neuropsichiatria Infantile. Several patients with epilepsy were incidentally observed to have CD, which prompted them to study epilepsy patients. Accidental discoveries often lead to incredible findings.

Only 2 had any gastro symptoms, though "most patients had recurrent diarrhoea, anaemia, and other symptoms suggestive of CD in the first 3 years of life.... The epilepsy in CEC [cerebral calcifications] patients was poorly responsive to antiepileptic drugs. Gluten-free diet beneficially affected the course of epilepsy only when started soon after epilepsy onset."[176] They suggest screening all epilepsy and cerebral calcification patients for CD.

Notice how often unchecked symptoms can lead to irreversible damage. Diarrhea and anemia could have led to faster diagnoses and less damage, but they were obviously considered "normal" and dismissed. Those kids could have been spared from epilepsy.

GLUTEN INDUCED SOCIAL PHOBIAS

Quality of Life is as subjective as art. Would you consider lifelong social phobias to be a problem? Not dementia, not seizures, but something that can easily fly under the radar and "Oh, Emily is just shy". What if Emily isn't shy and she was meant to do grand things in life, but the antibodies in her blood shot to her brain and held her back. Remember the Scandinavian study, showing an alarmingly higher number of low achievers with Celiac Disease, when all other factors were the same. Well...

"...a significantly higher prevalence of social phobia in CD patients compared with in healthy subjects. Future studies are needed to clarify the possible social phobia-induced risks such as school and/or work failure in CD patients."[177]

Would you consider lifelong social phobias to have a degenerative effect on someone's life experience? Career choices, who and if they marry, ...

"THIS IS ALL INSANE"

How many times have you thought, "What is all this? Brain lesions and heroin hits? It's insane!"

...Yes, *I know.* When I say the facts keep me up at night, just remember that I've got a little over 9,000 studies floating in my head (new kind of glutened brain). I committed to including only 300 in this book *(I went a little over, sorry)* so I wouldn't glutenize your brain too. You should see what happens to your heart after hugging a trembling 6-year-old that could have been saved if they were diagnosed before seizure-causing and mind-altering drugs damaged them irreversibly.

These foods are hitting people from all angles, and in varied ways. Several types of harmful proteins, gliadins, exorphins, opioids, ... infecting blood, brain, organs, ... pure chaos. And we've measured it all in scientific labs, there's no question to the damage. So why aren't we fixing it? I have no idea, *you tell me.*

Exorphins aren't exclusive to gluten, the same thing can happen with casein (dairy), causing (or worsening):
-Migraine[178]
-Bi-polar[179]
-Bi-polar[180] (with psychosis/mania)
-Schizophrenia[181]
-Autism[182]

Please note some of these studies also identified wheat gluten as causing or worsening these disorders. I'm showing you the higher end of the scale instead of mood swings or depression, simply to show how severely people react to casein.

The Division of Preventive Medicine, Walter Reed Army Institute of Research studied 855 U.S. soldiers discharged for schizophrenia and found elevated antibodies (IgG) to casein. "This is the first report to identify an association between the risk of schizophrenia and elevated antibodies to bovine casein prior to disease onset."[183]

...Let me guess: *But they're soldiers, very stressful, maybe it's not the casein.* Okay, I'll entertain that. Let's switch back to civilians without war stress. Come with me to Johns Hopkins University School of Medicine, Stanley Division of Developmental Neurovirology, Department of Pediatrics to look at onset psychosis and schizophrenia: "The elevated IgG and unique patterns of antibody specificity to bovine casein among diagnostic groups provide a rationale for clinical trials to evaluate efficacies of dietary modifications in individuals with neuropsychiatric diseases."[184]

Any other questions? I promise you solid, objective answers by the most credible sources. Yes, this stuff makes me swear in 5 languages and even speak in tongues sometimes, but my focus never comes off the facts. I geek first, rant second.

Now here's my zillion dollar question: Why? Why would anyone play on the highway with trucks zooming up and down, when there are completely safe places to play...

SOLUTIONS, HEALTHY ALTERNATIVES TO CASEIN

-Coconut milk
-Almond milk
-Cashew milk
-Hazelnut milk
-Hemp milk
-Flax milk
-Quinoa milk, ...

And unlike cow's milk, there are no cows involved *(I was this sarcastic by age 5, be grateful you weren't my parents, but notice there's truth/fact to everything I say).*

No cows means:
A) Less methane for the environment, which is on the verge of exploding
B) No imprisonment / mistreatment / medication of the poor animals
C) Less brain damage for humans

What's the downside here? Why do we need cow's milk when we have a dozen safe and more nutritious alternatives? What am I missing? Even cows stop drinking milk as soon as they develop teeth and can chew grass (all healthy roads lead back to greens).

I'm a moderately intelligent person, someone explain to me the up side of eating foods we've proven cause brain damage. I'm open and listening.

F.A.Q. "WHAT ABOUT CALCIUM AND OSTEOPOROSIS?"

A: What about it? The countries that eat/drink the most dairy are the ones with the highest levels of osteoporosis (US, UK, Finland, Sweden). Per capita, Norway is highest in osteoporosis, and it's a high dairy-consuming country.

The Western World and Europe consume a lot of dairy and suffer higher levels of osteoporosis compared to Asia and Africa, where they did not consume much dairy until recently. As the Western food habits of gluten and dairy make their way East, Asia and Africa are beginning to suffer from the same diseases, including higher levels of psychosis and osteoporosis.[185]

The same way dental journals and associations have pointed out the overwhelming link of dental decay with gluten, so have journals regarding bone health. Like the dental journals, internal medicine suggests immediate screening for Celiac Disease when a patient comes in with osteoporosis.[186] Hip fractures with CD are more common as well.[187] Columbia University did a presentation specifically on this at a Digestive Conference in Orlando.[188]

Forget the white mustaches of Hollywood stars brought to you by the trillion-dollar dairy industry. *Another 900 points to the Marketing Masters.* Watch stars for entertainment, listen to geeks for information. When you want computer programming advice, you go to Bill Gates, not Daniel Craig, even though 007 is sexier.

NON-SCHIZOPHRENIC-INDUCING SOURCES OF CALCIUM:

Sesame seeds (tahini), chia seeds, almonds (raw nut butters maintain their nutritional value), Brazil nuts, hazelnuts, pistachios, walnuts, dried figs, sunflower seeds, flax seed, seaweed, kale, leeks, collards, dandelion, parsley, mustard greens, celery, broccoli, brussel sprouts, watercress, even oranges have calcium... and none of these create antibodies in your system.

Once again, all roads lead back to green. Where do you think the cow is getting its calcium from?? It's time to cut out the middleman and go straight to the (usually green) source.

Legally GF Doesn't Mean Actually GF

GRAS: Generally Regarded As Safe

One of many legal technicalities that allows toxic food to be labeled as safe. What does "generally" mean? It means it didn't kill the majority of people in a study. ...Unless they got hospitalized and were forced to drop out of the study before it finished, in that case, they weren't considered in the conclusion at all.

WHEN LEGAL LOOPHOLES CAUSE BRAIN DAMAGE...

I tear apart studies and question how laws are being set on everything. It's long, tedious, boring, can be upsetting, and I totally understand why you wouldn't want to do it. Please go through it once with me, on one food, so that you'll understand how the current laws are hurting you.

This could also be the answer to: "I buy everything gluten-free, why don't I still feel well?" (you're not alone, most people don't feel fantastic, even though they think they're gluten free)

OATS

As of 2017, oats are no longer considered gluten-free by Health Canada (They listed oats as GF for decades... so in a few decades, what other foods will get scratched off today's "safe" list?)

This is a good example of:

1) There isn't a 100% consensus on what's GF or not

2) Countries keep playing catch-up to each other (no country has it all perfectly right, though Australia is the leader for sure)

For a long time, the media has been repeating that oats are fine, "it's just the cross-contamination factor, handling in transport, sharing same production lines as flour mills, etc." They said it again and again, to the point where oat companies took it upon themselves to put "gluten-free oats" on the front of their packages. Zero science, all marketing.

Even when ensured to not be contaminated by other products, carefully contained in a science lab, "oats do affect the gut microflora function."[189] If it impacts the gut, it'll impact the brain.

Some studies show that Celiacs were able to tolerate oats... *What does that mean?* "Able to tolerate" means there wasn't blood in their stool or immediate adverse reactions that required hospitalization.

...You probably think I'm being sarcastic... *I wish I was.* There have been studies trying to measure "acceptable gluten intake" where patients had to drop out due to severe reactions, including hospitalization and blood in stool[190] ...That was on 10mg of gluten, which is the equivalent of 0.002 teaspoon.

The result of that study? That more studies were needed to determine what the majority of Celiac patients can tolerate. I see those things and don't even know where to start ranting. As long as several people got severely sick, why are we even still questioning whether those foods should be labeled safe? What's there to measure? If 0.002 teaspoon can put Gluten Sensitive people in the hospital, then it's not safe. End of story. Of course, that simplistic thinking is bad for ale. Instead, let's measure how much (most) people can eat without immediately bleeding...

"The majority of patients with coeliac disease could consume up to 100 g/d of uncontaminated oats"[191]

1) "The majority of patients", not everyone. This is where GRAS kicks in. And they're just talking outwardly symptoms.

2) "Up to 100 g/d" ...and then what happens? This study never specified how sick people got when they consumed more than 100g (or whatever the number, depending on the study). Are they going to stand in your kitchen and measure 100g out for you? *Are you?* If you have a box of those cookies in your house, you're going to control your 5-year-old and make sure they don't eat more than half a cookie per day? Why would you do that if you can give them unlimited almond or coconut or a long list of other completely safe cookies?

No one even sees those limitations, there's no legal requirement to state them on the packaging. Have you ever seen a granola box that says "Gluten-Free Oats, but if you have Celiac/NCGS, eat less than 100 grams per day", or if it's an energy bar: "Celiac customers be sure to eat less than 3/4 of one bar per day, if there's blood in your stool, it'll usually heal within 3-6 months, and then you can resume eating our product". Of course not. All you see is "Certified Gluten-Free Oats" and guess where those certifications are coming from? Not government. They're coming from self-created, self-regulated, gluten certification offices.

So now we have this happy network of Celiac Associations supporting non-regulated Gluten Certification Businesses and commending them for supporting the Celiac Community. RN's are hired to implement the programs, because "registered" anything looks good... (I'm not criticizing nurses, their intentions are good. I personally think nurses should be paid quadruple what they are, bless them, I could never do their job.)

So, between self-declared governance of Certified GF and Celiac Associations, everyone's holding hands and singing songs around a campfire while toasting sugar-loaded, toxic, certified gluten-free marshmallows, meanwhile, no one is actually looking at the science.

No one is questioning why the long-term wellness of people with Celiac Disease is still poor, even when they are on strict gluten free diets. I am. *Please Keep Reading...*

Grains Deconstructed

If you thought the oat fiasco was bad, say hello to the corn fiasco because it's even worse (don't shoot the messenger). Note to parts of the world that refer to several foods as "corn": On this page and throughout this book, corn is referring exclusively to maize, otherwise I say "grain".

In 2009 I published (online articles and in books) studies showing people getting quite sick with exposure to maize. Here's what I posted:

This study goes back to 1979, showing 44% of people with Celiac Disease reacting negatively to corn. And it's not just people with CD that corn creates negative reactions in the gut for, it's also affecting people with several other disorders involving the gut: "Antibodies to Maize in Patients with Crohn's Disease, Ulcerative Colitis and Celiac Disease."[192]

And another study showing harmful antibodies to not only wheat gluten, but also: "wheat glutenins, albumins, and globulins, as well as against barley, oats, and maize prolamines."[193]

I posted nothing but facts and that was the 2nd highest amount of hate mail I received regarding "how wrong I was". I had to hire an assistant to manage my inbox for months. ...And yet, all I was doing was reporting facts from several studies, adding no personal opinion of my own. People with CD were becoming so violently ill eating the gluten of corn, they were forced to drop out of studies, which seemed like significant information that all Celiacs should know. Immediately, I saw this was hitting a terrible nerve for a lot of people.

When someone has a food restriction like gluten, the last thing they want is another food restriction. It's even worse to suggest corn could be an issue because corn is the default go-to when wheat is taken away. If you take away corn, you take away most processed foods, right down to bouillon cubes. To cook and take control of food again is unfathomable to most people, our lifestyle just isn't designed that way anymore. Our overall food habits are wound up around grains, so to remove grains altogether can seem impossible (notice how grains are holding people hostage, we've become enslaved to one food).

Most people can't even process the suggestion, they'll immediately say: "But what will I eat? Just meat and vegetables? How will I feel full?" We'll get to solutions shortly, first, understand the problem and why you might want to remove all grains from your plate, whether you think you're Gluten Sensitive or not...

Those studies I originally wrote about were all measuring gut damage or symptoms that immediately rose, they weren't measuring long term damage as far as creating malnutrition or brain damage. Corn does hit your brain and will create mood disorders, though I'm not sure how many studies titled "Corn malnutrition, brain serotonin and behavior"[194] we'll see anymore. That was 1976, before food and chemical companies really started flexing their muscles in public. When you can sue Oprah Winfrey for making a personal comment on her own show, you're going to silence a lot of people and scientists aren't going to be too eager to put themselves in that kind of line of fire. If you think the meat industry has power, you haven't met the Grain Cartel yet. *Good thing Oprah only mentioned the burger and not the bun.*

Did you know it's illegal (so far, in 13 states) to say anything that can affect sales of food? It's called Food Libel Laws (or food disparagement laws). The Be-Quiet-Law isn't just stateside. Britain had a case[195] that dragged out for 10 years: McDonald's suing two environmental activists who put out a pamphlet about them (food poisoning as well as overtime issues with employees and environmental concerns). McDonald's threw millions of dollars at the case, and the defendants could afford almost nothing, relied on pro bono help after being denied public defenders. Not such a happy meal to lose 10 years of your life for printing things that were never dis-proven. The only reason the case even ended at 10 years is because of bad press, they didn't want to look like McGoliath crushing the little Davids for decades. Messy case all around.

I'm not sure where Freedom of Speech belongs in all this, but I can tell you most people don't feel free to speak, so you're not going to hear a lot of criticism about corn. Note to Grain Cartel: I'm only reporting facts and quoting studies previously published by hospitals, universities, and research centers.

NOT JUST GLUTEN, IT'S ALL COMPONENTS OF ALL GRAINS

PHYTIC ACID (also called phytates): Are nature's built-in pest control devices for insects and rodents to stay away from grains (so the seed can grow and provide real food). Most animals smell it and stay away. Humans add yet more chemicals.

-Brain of flees: 10
-Brain of humans: 0

Sarcasm aside, there are serious nutrient deficiencies caused by phytic acid[196]. Zinc and iron[197] are common, but not exclusive.

WHEAT GERM AGGLUTININ: Another natural toxin to protect the grain. WGA does direct damage to the gut.[198] It eats away at your microvilli (whose job is to absorb nutrients, kill the villi and how will your body absorb nutrients anymore?)

WGA is 100% indigestible, you can't cook it out, can't steam, bake, grill, or exorcise it out with a priest. WGA itself is indestructible, but it destroys whatever crosses its path.

WGA also instantly affects the platelets[199] in your blood, which means it instantly hits your entire body. "WGA, which is a very potent platelet stimulator, elicited a rapid surge in Syk."[200] You're thinking, *what does Syk mean to me?* "The central role played by Syk [spleen tyrosine kinase] in the immune system in mediating inflammatory responses."[201] Wheat is weakening your system in ways you can't imagine. When you compromise Syk, you're compromising your body's ability to deal with inflammation. So now you're setting off the chain reaction to open yourself up to inflammatory related disorders, crippling arthritis being one of them.

YOU CAN'T COOK OR FERMENT WGA OUT

Special note to the sourdough/fermentation team grasping at straws: You can't ferment harm out. Finland loves their bread as much as you do, Helsinki did a study, not even with Celiac Disease but with Wheat Sensitive people and Irritable Bowel Syndrome: "the sourdough bread was not tolerated better than the yeast-fermented bread."[202] (that's regarding gluten, not just WGA)

...That topic was the highest amount of hate mail I got, when I said fermented isn't better, even though Michael Pollan (who I adore and am a big fan of) did a little no-no in his documentary "Cooked" and suggested fermented was fine for all. He's a great guy (professor of journalism and a botanist, never read a single scientific thing about CD, now author and star), but he didn't have a single expert there, wasn't even pronouncing "Celiac" correctly. I'm not an English teacher, I don't care if he pronounced it right or wrong, I'm just saying if he had a single expert on the topic consult him, he would have been saying it right - it's like a Poker tell when they pronounce it wrong. His expert was an ex-tech guy mocking GF and saying there's "no proof" of gluten doing harm (somebody please get him this book), and a third generation baker who knows nothing about CD/NCGS, might never even of heard of them, he just knows how to bake (Note to Producers: nice touch getting a dude with a French accent, even though he's from Quebec and not France. Next time, maybe a little attention to accuracy on a disorder that can debilitate? Merci)

P.S. Mr. No-Proof-of-Gluten-Being-Harmful is producing a line of gluten free food. He might not understand the topic, but he certainly understands profit and a growing market.

They would never do that with diabetes or any other disease, they would bring on true experts. CD is treated very differently from every other disorder, which is why people resist testing so much, they can't bear the thought of becoming the kid in the schoolyard that will be mocked every day for the rest of their lives. It's a tough gig.

ALPHA-AMYLASE INHIBITORS: Spain did an interesting study[203] focused on NCGS with wheat and other cereals, "appear as potential activator of innate immunity in NCGS patients." Yet another non-gluten component of wheat that's damaging health.

Germany: "ATIs may be prime candidates of severe forms of non-celiac gluten (wheat) sensitivity."[204]

"Gluten-containing cereals have by far the highest concentrations of ATIs that activate TLR4. Orally ingested ATIs are largely resistant to proteases and heat, and increase intestinal inflammation by activating gut and mesenteric lymph node myeloid cells."[205]

...More medical jargon, let me simplify: Myeloid cells affect bone marrow and spine. Don't invite Leukemia into your life, it's not a guest you can easily get rid of.

"Wheat amylase trypsin inhibitors drive intestinal inflammation... may fuel inflammation and immune reactions in other intestinal and nonintestinal immune disorders."[206]

We've known for decades that gluten can cause health issues. Then scientists discover amylase from wheat causes inflammation.[207] Lately they've identified fructans[208] from wheat are a problem and also exacerbate IBS symptoms.[209]

IBS SIDE NOTE: The medical community is starting to acknowledge that IBS is highly affected by wheat and that many IBS patients are misdiagnosed, they are actually CD or NCGS patients. I'll make just one quick reference[210], their IBS patients:
1) 34% had measurable Wheat Sensitivity
2) 52% had genes for Celiac Disease
3) At 1-year follow up, ALL improved gluten-free

UNDISCOVERED COMPONENTS

The above are some of the harmful components we know about, but there are still components we don't know about (who knew so much can be wrapped up in one little grain?)

While looking for the cause of NCGS, Netherlands study: "Its pathogenesis remains obscure but may be related to non-gliadin molecules in grains that stimulate the innate immune system of the intestine."[211]

Molecules unrelated to gluten and gliadin will still be discovered in the coming years.

I can keep going, but is there a need to? Are you getting a sense of the volumes and volumes of data? Every single page that's got any technical/medical element to it can be a book of its own, and I still wouldn't be able to fit all the scientific data in a reasonable length of book.

All grains create issues. Some more than others, but none of them can be classified as healthy and none of them have any unique nutrients that you can't find in plant food.

RICE is the least powerful gangster in the streets, but it still does damage. Potentially serious damage, like Enterocolitis Syndrome in children.[212] That said, experience has taught me most people can't make the jump to completely grain free instantly... even I didn't let go of rice in the beginning *(until I saw Enterocolitis Syndrome).*

If you're eating rice, get your hands on ancient rice, it doesn't seem to create the same havoc as modern rice.[213] Make sure it's organic, and remember the natural arsenic element, so it's not something you want to eat daily.

To wrap up on a good note, scientists are finding "a novel neurological function of rice bran". It seems it affects sleep and "could be a promising therapeutic agent for insomnia."[214] *Zzzzzzz...* at least we can dream about better health in deep sleep ;)

TICKING TIME BOMBS

The thing about inflammation, and autoimmune disorders, is that you have no idea when the bomb will go off. Once it does, you have no idea what you'll find in the remains. Sometimes you can rebuild, sometimes you can't. I can't undo 21 root canals. The Dentistry Association in Michigan said: "Appropriate referral and a timely diagnosis can help prevent serious complications of this disorder."[215] [referring to CD]

Those "serious complications" extend far beyond things we can x-ray in a dentist's chair. Less tangibly, I can't undo the life cost of being a hot-tempered person and thinking it was hereditary. *"You're a hot head, just like your father,"* cost me work, putting my professional life on a different trajectory. It cost me relationships, putting my personal life on a different trajectory. It turns out I'm Zen calm. ...That took 8 months of being GF to discover. I was almost 40 before I knew my own temperament. I had to get reacquainted with myself and adjust to a person I wasn't familiar with. Better person, but unfamiliar. My "hereditary hot temper" could have easily gone further up the scale, to more violent and destructive behavior. Then what?

The neuropsychiatric impact of gluten is its most terrorizing effect. Hyper symptoms can disappear quickly, what takes time is the full brain regeneration (and that's if you're feeding it right). Eating gluten is like a severe alcoholic who always has alcohol in their blood. It's constantly altering their blood, brain, emotions, and behavior. Gluten has the same effect. It's always invisibly there, doing its thing, and you're so used to it, you'll never realize it's there until you become sober and stay sober long enough for your entire body to rid itself of all traces. For me, that was almost a year, even though I looked and felt physically fine within 90 days.

The question is: Why play with a ticking time bomb? That's a sincere question. I have yet to hear any answer that makes sense to me. Why jog in a land mine and risk losing a limb if you can jog on a safe path? What's the reason? It tastes better? Step into my kitchen, I challenge any food you bring me with a purer version.

Someone took me up on that challenge with Tiramisu. Italian dude (he'd shoot me for saying that, pardon L, Sicilian dude... *there's a difference you know* ;) He was the bartender at the wood burning stove pizza place I used to go to every Friday night pre-Celiac.

We became buddies and stayed friends after Celiac (he cried out loud when he got my news). I made a raw version of Tiramisu and brought it to his next party. He took a bite, walked over to me, dropped to his knees, kissed my hand, and hasn't called me by my name since. ...The trick is explaining what "Raw Goddess" means to bartenders and waiters every time we're out together :) ...And his best friend calls me every 6 months to propose, with the condition I make raw cake every weekend. Both sworn gluten and sugar addicts, ejected from the womb with a Cannoli already in their mouths.

It comes down to commitment and either learning how to make better food or finding places that do. The options are all there in most cities. Sometimes it's a question of getting a bread loaf from this shelf instead of that one or walking 15 feet over to the frozen aisle and getting gluten-free bread (though that'll still mean you're eating grains, but getting off gluten is still a good halfway point). The convenience factor is the same.

It'll cost more, but most people can make up for the difference in cost just by eating out a few less times per year. See two less movies at the cinema, buy one less piece of clothing that you're barely going to wear. I discuss priorities with people before I discuss details and food plans. If you have CD, chances are you're eating out a whole lot less, so re-direct that money to higher quality groceries.

POWER TIP: When you begin the transition to real food (especially if you get off all grains), you'll get the illusion of feeling hungry all the time, even five minutes after eating. You're not hungry. You're simply not used to feeling light and energetic after meals. Your body (probably since being a toddler) has been conditioned to work really, really hard to process the cement bricks you keep sending it to digest. When you send it pure food, it knows exactly what to do with it, processes quickly and easily, and is free quickly. Free to... do anything... be, go, run, walk, play, love, kiss, hug,... *to l.i.v.e.*

You'll get used to the light feeling and wonder how it was possible you got through life before. Once you're aware this will happen for a few weeks, you'll be able to handle it easily instead of what many do, which is say (on day 1 or 2): *"This doesn't work for me, I need more solid foods."* No. You don't. You need to get back to eating to live, not eating to fall into lethargy and brain fog.

Know it's going to happen, laugh when it does, *"Aha, Jaqui said I'd feel deceivingly hungry at first,"* and let it pass. Wait it out, it *will* pass, and then you'll get your life back. Down a tall glass or two of water every time it happens, it'll help that deceiving feeling of hunger.

Sugar

When it comes to sugar, for the longest time, the sole focus was obesity. Yes, sugar does make you fat, but there's more to it than that. Sugar creates inflammation in your brain and chemically stresses you.

"The overconsumption of fructose, which leads to inflammation in all cells that metabolize it rapidly... fructose in the brain... stimulates an increased release of cortisol."[216]

Cortisol isn't supposed to be floating in your bloodstream unless your life is in imminent danger. It shouldn't be there because you ate what you thought was a healthy energy bar.

The hippocampus is the part of your brain that affects emotions, memory, and more. Fructose directly damages (well, *everything,* but I'll stick to the focus of this particular study) the hippocampus and creates oxidization (rusting) in the brain.

"The fructose-induced inflammatory condition was associated with brain oxidative stress... In conclusion, these results suggest that unbalanced diet, rich in fructose, may be highly deleterious in young people as in adults and must be strongly discouraged for the prevention of diet-associated neuroinflammation and neurological diseases."[217]

That's not an isolated study showing damage to the brain, this one[218] showed hippocampus damage with 9 weeks of high fructose intake. 9 weeks. What happens after 20 years? 50 years?

They can measure brain inflammation as well as direct damage to specific regions, like the hippocampus. We also know that high sugar causes insulin resistance. That's a brain problem because you need insulin to increase in order to trigger communications. Your brain is lethargic without insulin.

That lethargy, brain fog, is so common now, you hear people laughingly refer to themselves: *"Yeah, I know I'm ADHD".* When a brain disorder gets accepted as a norm in culture and even appears in pop songs, we need to have a collective discussion.

"I'm trying to focus my attention
But I feel so A.D.D.
I need some help some inspiration
But it's not coming easily"
-Natasha Bedingfield, "These Words" (awesome tune)

...Not so entertaining if it graduates to dementia and she can't remember the words to her song.

Sugar also triggers dopamine, making it as addictive as narcotics. The sugar rush you're getting (not to be mistaken for energy) shoots serotonin up, makes you happy for 20 minutes, then drops like a bomb. So you go back for more, more, more. No different from crack.

A client once said to me: "I can't stop eating sugar, I've tried before and it makes me feel horrific. I immediately become anxious, depressed, my brain gets mushy and I get so very sad."

My response: "Doesn't that frighten you? Don't you think it's a slave-master you need to free yourself from?"

She was so desperate for me to say she can have some artificial sugar, that she went to her Weight Watchers mentor, who told her I was being too strict and pointed her to a study that said it's prudent to have sugar in moderation. Prudent? To eat sugar? I looked into that study[219] and found:

"Conflict of interest statement: J.M. Rippe's research laboratory has received unrestricted grants and J.M. Rippe has received consulting fees from ConAgra Foods, Kraft Foods, the Florida Department of Citrus, PepsiCo International, The Coca Cola Company, the Corn Refiners Association, Weight Watchers International and various publishers."

"Unrestricted grants", gotta love them. How do we fight an industry with more money than God? How do we fight an industry that can sue God and win?

It's challenging to see people need a sugar fix as bad as narcotic addicts. That sugar fix makes you more insulin-resistant, makes your gut more permeable, hits your liver, makes you fatter faster, ages you, oxidizes your brain, creates full body inflammation as well as brain-specific inflammation[220] ...*I think I can stop now.*

While sugar has 90 commercial names it runs under, the most common you'll see are:
-High-Fructose Corn Syrup
-Fructose
-Glucose
-Dextrose
-Cane Sugar (Don't let the word cane fool you, 500 more points to the Marketing Masters, where do you think sugar was coming from before?)

Get used to breaking things down, you need to start seeing food with my eyes. How does cane sugar differ from any other processed white sugar? Sugar canes are natural only if you're chewing on the canes themselves, not processed white stuff made from sugar canes. FYI sugar canes are green outside and look like thin bamboo shoots. Your jaws would get tired of chewing before brain damage happened. *Yet again, green is good, even when it comes to sugar.*

Have you ever examined the food labels of nourishment and energy bars? I fall into glycemic shock just looking at them. Ignore the words "healthy", "enriched", "vitamin this", "mineral that" on the front of the package. Also ignore the athletes' pictures. Please become completely blind to the front of the package. Read the ingredients labels in tiny print and bring an adding machine with you to count how many sugars are there. Most "healthy bars" cause brain damage, disrupt your thyroid, wreck your insulin, and make you fat. While they still need to print ingredients lists (I'm sure it's legally in the works to remove that pesky part of packaging), get in the habit of checking labels.

Natural Sweeteners

Anaheim, California. I'm at a conference for food industry professionals, before the bigger conference to consumers opens up days later. The speakers are two lawyers, discussing the word "natural" as it relates to food labels and how the FDA is unable to release a statement with a clear definition, and how food companies can use the word natural without getting in trouble.

I always get an ice-cream-brain-freeze effect with these things. Natural. How complicated is it? Since governments, lawyers, biologists, chemists, food science PhD's, food company CEO's can't define it (that's who was in the room in California), why don't I humbly give it a try: "Food from the earth, unadulterated by humans". Is that a definition we can all agree on?

There are many aspects to our sci-fi food world that are very much about hiding things in plain sight. "Natural Sweeteners" is one of them. Did you know that stevia is up to 300 times more condensed than sugar? The long list of natural sweeteners is starting to rival the list of unnatural sweeteners. It took 70 years to admit what refined sugar and high-fructose corn syrup and all the other *oses* and *exes* do to your brain (dexTROSE, frucTOSE ... their ending gives them away). And in 50-60-70 years they'll have enough human experiments and studies to tell you what these processed natural sweeteners are doing to you (ask for WIFI in your coffin).

STEVIA (I don't mean to be singling it out, it's simply the example I'm using, apply this info across the board with all sweeteners)

There are a lot of studies regarding the benefits of the stevia leaf. The leaf. *The Green Leaf.* The reason I'm not bringing them to you: You're not chewing on the fresh green leaf (it looks like mint).

Stevia is like Cocaine: When you take the leaf from the jungle and chew it, it's natural and harmless, may even be beneficial. When you take the leaf and process it into a white powder, like cocaine, it's not so harmless anymore. You're giving your body a massive jolt (not the sexy kind of jolt like meeting Jason Momoa or Vin Diesel). You're making your cells scramble and run for dear life, except they're trapped, there's nowhere to go. They have no choice but to sit in your body and get jolted for all the wrong reasons. Shock them enough times and they get fried, malfunction, struggle, send you cries for help (called symptoms, which your MD will happily silence), go on life support, then die prematurely.

We're slowly getting question marks: "Sweeteners are highly chemically diverse including natural sugars, sugar alcohols, natural and synthetic sweeteners... The accumulated knowledge on sugar substitutes raises the issue of potential health effects."[221]

Stevia isn't hanging out with green buddies: "(aspartame, saccharine, sucralose, neotame, acesulfame-K, and stevia) have previously received a generally recognized as safe status from the United States Food and Drug Administration...

...there is inconclusive evidence to support most of their uses and some recent studies even hint that these earlier established benefits regarding NNS (Nonnutritive sweeteners) use might not be true.

...Pregnant and lactating women, children, diabetics, migraine, and epilepsy patients represent the susceptible population to the adverse effects of NNS-containing products and should use these products with utmost caution. The overall use of NNS remains controversial, and consumers should be amply informed about the potential risks of using them."[222]

But the Stevia money train took off a while ago. Companies are in place, distribution is widespread, it's in tens of thousands of commercial recipes (the cost of changing recipes for agri-food is massive, not something they do often, regardless of what they discover about an ingredient). Stevia is here to stay because it's already been worked into The Modern Food Matrix.

HOW THESE SWEETENERS WORK

They trigger your taste receptors (T1R2/T1R3). When you jolt your taste receptors with unnatural levels of sweetness, you alter them. Any time you alter a natural process, there are repercussions. When you alter your natural palate, real food won't taste good to you because it hasn't been sweetened like your "healthy granola bar" with its natural sweeteners and "healthy protein shake" with its 300x sweetener.

These "natural sweeteners" (that you need lawyers, lobbyists, biologists, engineers, and a chemical processing plant to create), make it hard for your own receptors to enjoy pure food. The myth is that receptors are only in the mouth/tongue. No, no, no... "In the gut, this receptor has been suggested to be involved in luminal glucose sensing, the release of some satiety hormones, the expression of glucose transporters, and the maintenance of glucose homeostasis."[223]

Let me break that down for you:
1) **"Glucose sensing"** is not something we want to trick. Tricking it is inviting malfunction down the road.
2) **"Satiety hormones"** getting artificially triggered can A) Create addiction/craving to that item. B) Misfire and tell you that you need more food, making you eat more. Great for the food manufacturer, not so great for your bikini body and foggy brain.
3) **"Glucose homeostasis"** is a happy place and not a state you want to disrupt. Don't mess with glucose and insulin levels, that's not a war you'll ever win.

...I'm sure there are even more issues that I'm not scientifically smart enough to identify. What I do know: Mess with your natural state and bad things happen. That sounds vague, doesn't it? Like I'm guessing? Never. I don't mess around when it comes to people being sick. Here's another study including "natural sweeteners" and the title says it all: "What Does Diabetes "Taste" Like?"...

..."Importantly, the T1R2/T1R3 sweet taste receptor is also expressed in extra-oral tissues, including the stomach, pancreas, gut, liver, **and brain**. Although its physiological role remains to be established in numerous organs, T1R2/T1R3 is suspected to be involved in the **regulation of metabolic processes**, such as sugar sensing, glucose homeostasis, and **satiety hormone** release. In this review, the physiological role of the sweet taste receptor in taste perception and metabolic regulation is discussed by focusing on **dysfunctions leading to diabetes**."[224]

"Dysfunctions leading to diabetes" ... No, thank you. I'm fine with dates or maple syrup when I need something extra sweet, rare as that is.

The problem isn't just diabetes, it's brain malfunction. It's the glycation process of sugar on cells in your brain and body. Glycation is the hardening element, think crème brûlée and that hardened surface, or like when bread bakes and the outside gets hard.

When sugar sticks to your brain molecules, and hardens, that's the same glycation as crème brûlée. Glycation on your cells is irreversible, you can't un-bake bread. The molecule can't breathe, move, communicate... it can't do its job. It suffocates and dies. Kill enough brain molecules and you have brain damage. Kill some more, and you can't remember your own name. That kind of brain degeneration is how we get to severe dementia. All this, to artificially sweeten a "healthy smoothie".

Q: "What if I can't deal with an unsweetened smoothie? I just can't. It's too awful tasting and I end up not having one at all. I need my delicious protein shake or I won't do it."

A: I get it. I truly, technically, get it, more precisely than you can imagine. There's scientific proof of what happens when taste receptors are altered, so I completely believe an unsweetened smoothie feels unbearable to you. I've got you covered...

4 SWEET SOLUTIONS
(apply the same to cakes, cookies, and anything else you sweeten)

1) **DATES.** Sweet, easy to have on hand since they store a long time, and versatile (I use them for the base of cheesecakes or recipes that need something sticky, not just sweet). Your body uses dates as natural fuel, a little more suited to marathon running than everyday life, but we'll go with it :) (Don't ever say I'm totally inflexible)

2) **BANANAS.** The riper they are, the sweeter they are. I can't eat them once the little black spots appear, but I can make banana bread with them. Cut them up into cubes and freeze them, add to your smoothie. They'll provide sweetness as well as a creamy thick texture, and excellent nutrients.

3) **MAPLE SYRUP.** Lowest on the glycemic index and comes with some beneficial properties. So far, no one is adulterating maple syrup.

4) **HONEY.** Actually contains 2000 enzymes that don't exist anywhere else, it's as complex a food as cacao. Manuka honey (the higher the number, the more properties in it), is extra powerful.

There it is, 4 ways to naturally sweeten any food or drink, without any health risks (diabetes patients, apply your precautions of course). Each option actually comes with benefits, which is Standard Operating Procedure in the world of real, pure food.

Besides real fruit, the only exceptions to these might be some kind of sap that drips out of trees or plants in jungles I haven't been in and don't know about. If you encounter such sweets, get a picture next to the tribes-people that showed it to you, get a close-up of the (probably green) leaf, and send me both pictures along with an audio of what the indigenous people call it so we'll know how to pronounce it ;)

No processing, no machinery, no labs, no factories, no engineers, no biologists, no way it could have existed 1,000,000 years ago. That's how you know if you have a natural sweetener or not, and it shouldn't be in your life very often. Fruit contains all the sugar you can possibly ever need.

AGAVE: I get asked about it a lot and see a lot of raw food people using it. My answer is: I don't know, the science is inconclusive.[225] There might possibly even be benefits,[226] they're studying it for cancer issues. But there might also be harmful factors with serious elements that affect insulin resistance. And there have been no studies on how it affects taste receptors, satiety hormones... there are too many question marks for me. I'll keep my eye out for any new info. JK jury is out on agave as of this publishing.

THE QUESTION TO APPLY TO ALL FOOD

Whether we're talking sweeteners or any other food, here's the question to ask yourself: "If I was the first person on earth and had no tools or machinery, could I make this with my bare hands or things I could create with bare hands?"

Honey: Yes, you can stick your hand in after a colony is done and take their leftover honey (this is what an organic beekeeper does, they're not stealing baby bees' food, all bees make more than they need, leave it behind, start again). And organic means the poor little souls aren't getting sprayed, they're in their natural healthy happy state. Organic beekeepers adore and protect their bees (as I write this, several of them are refusing to take their bees to blueberry fields that have been spraying pesticides).

Maple Syrup: Yes, you can take a rock and poke a hole in a tree, then take a bamboo shoot and let the syrup drip into an empty coconut shell.

Sugar Cane: You can snap the green cane with bare hands and chew.

Dates: You can pick them off trees and eat, just like fruit.

Everything else: No way to make it with bare hands. Please stop jolting your poor little innocent cells and your brain. Just because you're holding them hostage in your body doesn't mean they don't deserve a peaceful existence.

Fish, Fish Oils, All Seafood

WARNING: You'll *definitely* want to tap out when you start reading this section. Please don't. For your brain health, I have to ask you to stay with me because...

As you look to do things to improve your brain health, every health expert and well-meaning holistic doctor in the world will tell you to eat "wild" fish. They'll usually specify salmon, and they'll suggest you take fish oil supplements too. Many of them sell their own private label brands of them.

insert foghorn Wild doesn't exist anymore. I'm about to give you the current science of our oceans and its inhabitants.

Know that my purpose isn't to overwhelm or upset you, it's to give you solid knowledge so that you make healthy decisions and you won't be affected by marketing or well-intentioned people who just aren't informed. It's not fun or easy reading (well, one part is), but if you want to protect your brain health, it's essential reading. I've broken it down into 4 parts (could have been way more) and I do give you omega-3 solutions. Here we go...

1) METALS AND CHEMICALS (MERCURY IS ONE OF MANY)

Whales in the Arctic are testing positive for cancer and artificial substances are being found in them. The Arctic, where no one exists, no industrial companies are based, no direct dumping is happening.

Quebec did a study on hundreds of beluga whales turning up dead in the St. Lawrence estuary. "The major primary causes of death were respiratory and gastrointestinal infections with metazoan parasites (22%), cancer (18%), and bacterial, viral, and protozoan infections (17%)"[227] (that was over 20 years ago, the toxic load is much worse now). **"Organic Wild Caught" fish come from those same waters.** Wild doesn't mean safe, not anymore. And notice mercury is nowhere on that report, we have more than one toxin to think about.

PAY ATTENTION: It can legally be labeled organic because the fisherman and fisheries don't add chemicals to the catch. It doesn't matter that the fish were born in and are loaded with chemicals and cancer, as long as the fishery doesn't manually add chemicals, it's organic (and wild caught).

San Francisco, California, 2018: 14 sampling stations were set up to collect water samples. I hope you're sitting for this… "Fecal pollution of surface waters presents a global human health threat… with detection frequency at some stations as high as 97%."[228]

Chemical dumping isn't the only issue with our oceans, human waste is as well. …When they tell you tuna and big fish in the ocean are bad, but smaller fish don't contain as much mercury and are better… *insert foghorn warning* Mercury isn't the only problem with seafood, and how does it make sense to have "less poison" anyways?

Vancouver, Canada (West Coast, Pacific) looks pretty and pristine, the license plates say "Beautiful British Columbia", and it is stunningly pretty. I called it home at one time and might again soon. They're constantly putting out beach safety reports because E. coli is a recurring problem. The first time I saw that in the morning paper, I had been stand-up paddling in The English Bay (downtown) for weeks. They warn surfers and swimmers to not swallow the water, but they don't warn anyone about eating the fish that's being "wild caught" or "sustainably farmed" right upstream.

FYI: It's not a question of there being no E. coli, it's a question of whether it's less than 200 E. coli bacteria per 100 mL of water. There's always some level of it in the water, they've just figured out what level sends people to emergency wards (or morgue) versus a mysterious tummy ache that goes away in a few days. So, a fish born and living in that its whole life… *you do the math.* I say "morgue" for accuracy, not dramatic effect. Every time there's an E. coli outbreak, a few dozen people die.

Throughout this book, count how many different things are deemed "safe" because they're low-grade toxic. Is anyone adding them all up? How many assaults can we simultaneously take before our health starts to fail? Maybe our body can handle a little poison from one thing (why would we want to?), but when you add up a little poison from everything you're eating, it's not so safe anymore. By the end of two meals and one snack, your toxic load is over the "safe" limit. Be conscious of "toxic load". Let's keep going…

Canadian Arctic and waters to Labrador (East Coast, Atlantic and North) (just a short boat ride north of Maine) 2018 findings: Mercury (THg), PCBs, PCB 153, DDTs, p,p'-DDE, CHLs, ClBz, PBDEs, and PFOS.[229] …These are the same waters that advertise "wild caught" lobster and a long list of "healthy organic" fish and seafood. The study notes that these toxic levels of pollutants are found in seals and polar bears (who aren't in the water 24/7), so imagine the fish that are in that water 24/7. Also note that many of these chemicals, like DDT, banned in the 1970's in most countries, don't just go away.

This might be a good time to point out that many of today's "safe" foods, chemicals, and medications, might not be so safe...

DDT, known to cause devastating health issues, wasn't seen that way when it was first commercialized. In fact, Paul Müller, the Swiss chemist who brought DDT to human use, was awarded the Nobel Prize in Physiology or Medicine 1948 "for his discovery of the high efficiency of DDT as a contact poison against several arthropods".[230] He meant well, he was trying to control typhus and malaria.

Some of today's chemists mean well, the rest aren't ready to be whistle blowers and lose their lives. My point is, the government calling something safe isn't exactly a credible source. Never has been. Smoking was "safe" for 60 years.

Back to the U.S.A., testing from Florida, New Jersey, Virginia, and New York, 3 years of monitoring: "Associated with fatal paralytic shellfish poisoning (PSP) in the Pacific but not known to be toxic in the western Atlantic, P. bahamense is an emerging public health threat."[231]

Interesting that the "emerging public health threat" isn't on the 6 o'clock news, but Prozac and Viagra are. Who's going to spend billions of advertising dollars advising you to not eat something? Who would profit from that? **Shout out to billionaires:** *You might want to buy one less jet a year and help your fellow humans, Seashell Girl here has limited resources.*

What do you think shrimp from the Gulf of Mexico contain? You don't need to guess, there are marine biologists issuing warning reports yearly about 275+ toxins found in every size and species of fish. Here's one of hundreds of issues from the west coast of Florida, into the east and up the Carolinas: "Neurotoxic Shellfish Poisoning is typically caused by ingesting bivalve shellfish (clams, oysters and mussels), contaminated with brevetoxins. ...symptoms of NSP include both gastrointestinal and neurological problems. The most frequently reported symptoms are nausea, vomiting, abdominal pain, and diarrhea. ...Of greater concern to most individuals are the neurological symptoms which may include paresthesia of the mouth, lips, tongue; peripheral tingling, partial limb paralysis, slurred speech, dizziness, ataxia and a general loss of coordination."[232]

Since most people don't immediately die, it's ...*say it with me...* "generally regarded as safe" and approved for sale. Only "partial limb paralysis", not full paralysis, it must be fine then. *Lord help me control my language and present the facts objectively with no R-Rated words.* Notice they were talking clams, oysters, and mussels, not big fish.

The focus is always on large fish, tuna, swordfish... but that's limited, negligent, dangerous information. The most recent examinations of fish as tiny as minnows[233] and even oysters[234] are finding "that oil composition, concentration, and exposure duration all affect molecular responses in exposed fish, and suggest that low-concentration exposures may result in sub-lethal adverse effects." Oh, just *sub*-lethal, not totally lethal yet, then that must be okay. Let's wait until humans are dropping dead in restaurants upon consumption. Apparently, airplane-sized whales floating up dead on shores isn't lethal enough yet. *Please Keep Reading, you're an absolute star for hanging in there...*

MERCURY

"Environmental mercury (Hg) contamination is an urgent global health threat."[235] ...Not so urgent I guess, they're still advertising "low mercury, safe for pregnant women" ... WTF does "low mercury" mean? Why would we do that to a fetus?? Why would we do that to the mother, or the rest of us? How did we become conditioned enough to find this acceptable? Low mercury? This one has less poison than that one, so eat this one? *Seriously?*

While the scientists do their 50-year circles of "Are mercury and Alzheimer's disease linked?"[236] before they make a definitive statement, you might want to choose to play safe.

Seeing things drives home the point better than reading a clip of a study, so I suggest you look up a video called "Mercury Rising". It comes from the bonus features of the brilliant, shocking, mind-blowing documentary "The Cove" and shows you exactly what mercury does to your system, and what it did to people in Minamata, Japan, when there was a mercury issue there.

Mercury didn't just hurt a few people, it was catastrophic: "Minamata disease: catastrophic poisoning due to a failed public health response."[237] They managed to get footage from the 1950's when this tragedy happened and included it in this short clip.

Also in the clip, the director (activist, humanitarian, environmentalist, and "Game Changer" – which happens to be the name of his latest movie), Louie Psihoyos asks his doctor what mercury does to humans. His doctor responds that it slowly takes away what it means to be human. A Mercurial Moment of Truth. You can find it for free, just Google "Mercury Rising The Cove", only 18 minutes, worth watching, I'd call it lifesaving. And while you're at it, buy "The Cove" and support these guys. Psihoyos and his crew are real-life James Bonds, risking their lives to expose truths we should all be aware of. Watch the movie, but then go back and watch the director's cut to truly appreciate what they did.

2) MICRO-PLASTICS

Fish, of all sizes, are being found with micro-plastics in them. Like humans, it starts off in their intestinal tract, then makes its way into liver and other organs, and disease inevitably follows.

"Observed effects of microplastics ingestion include (but are not necessarily limited to) intestinal blockage, physical damage, histopathological alterations in the intestines, change in behavior, change in lipid metabolism, and transfer to the liver."[238]

If your fish has plastic in it and you eat that fish, you have plastic in you. Now it's *your* intestinal tract and organs that need to deal with it. This is a problem with both sea fish and freshwater fish.[239]

I've found hundreds of studies and reports showing hazardous levels of toxicity in fish and all seafood, but I have yet to find one that shows safety. I can find reports that say "relatively safe" and "believed to be safe for consumption" and passed by the FDA with no serious testing... but I have yet to find one study showing a single healthy sardine found, anywhere in the world. Show me one, just one little healthy happy sardine is all I'm asking for.

It's a global problem, "Microplastics are being detected in freshwaters of Europe, North America, and Asia[240]", India[241], Singapore[242], Canada[243], Portugal[244], Qatar[245], Belgium[246], Germany[247]... there's no safe place in the world because we're one world. One set of water.

Think of lakes and rivers as arteries, all connected and flowing into the ocean, which breathes up into the air, to the mountains/land, and the flow continues. The pollutants that don't flow via waterways, the wind carries everywhere. World pollution is one, singular problem.

The Dutch did a freshwater study and found microplastics are making their way into the ocean, they found them in all 15 locations along the Dutch North Sea coast they sampled.

"...'microplastics', brings synthetic materials that are non-degradable and biologically incompatible into contact with ecosystems... Marine species are heavily exposed to plastic particles... species inhabiting the Dutch North Sea coast: filter-feeding mussels and oysters (species for human consumption) as well as other consumers in the marine food chain."[248]

"Biologically incompatible" should be concerning. By legal definition, these mussels, oysters, and other seafood would be considered wild caught and organic.

If you think you're safe because you live in a sleepy town in the country in a beautiful, idyllic place, think again: "Microplastics in the sediments of a UK urban lake... growing burden of evidence for microplastic ubiquity in all environments."[249]

Biologists are sounding alarms and calling fish and overall water issues an "emerging threat", while the rest of the world is focused on colorful packages that promise "better focus" and "brain boost" and "less mercury than other products".
Biologists: 0
Marketers: 900

There's yet another element to consider, besides what it's doing to fish: Plastic in freshwater means plastic in drinking water. ...If you feel like your brain's going to blow up with all this bad news, welcome to my world. I'm reading 6000% more studies than I bring you. *I take a lot of quiet walks.*

HANG IN THERE

I'm not trying to overwhelm you, and I'm sorry for how much I'm throwing at you here. But I refuse to water down and give you sub-information that'll achieve nothing but sub-health.

As I ask during the extra-intense moments in live seminars, I'll ask you now: Are you alright? If it becomes too much, take a break. Step away, go for a walk, remember that there are solutions to all this... then come back. You only need to learn all this information once, then you're set for life.

As for the solutions: Like everything else in life, it takes a little time to adjust in the beginning and then everything will become second nature.

Please Keep Reading... You don't want to miss out on my favorite part of this entire book, you'll see what I mean next...

3) GENETICALLY MODIFIED AND FARMED FISH

The first thing you need to do is stop thinking the word "sustainable" is good. It's bad. Very, very bad. Sustainable fish are horrific and they terrorize me into sleep-walking episodes.

The real definition of sustainable: A cool, sexy, lean-muscled dude sits on a big rock with his bare feet on mineral rich soil, grounding, connecting. He takes a dry stick and small rock, exercising his arms while creating a harpoon. Then he walks on rugged terrain, munching on greens he forages along the way, until he steps onto the positive ions of the beach. He jumps into the clean, iodine-rich ocean and gets more exercise and natural vitamin D from above, while he catches two disease-free, non-plasticized, unmodified, sustainable fish. They're older, swimming slower, *it was their time.* He brings this back into the jungle while absorbing more minerals from the soil under his feet and munches on the berries he finds along the way. As he walks, he spits out the seeds, which become the future non-glyphosated crops. Once home, he enjoys an electronic-free, cell-phone-less dinner with his family, followed by an entertaining evening of story, song, and dance with others from the tribe. The moon is disappearing, fire down to embers, it's time for a pleasurable, non-Viagra-induced dance in the privacy of his tepee with his happy, healthy, non-Prozaced wife, after they put their unmedicated, athletic kids to sleep. *That* is sustainable. The fish they ate is sustainable.

...and then there were fish tanks (nets are the same problem)

Here's the definition of modern, genius-marketing, sustainable fish: 1) Salmon that are supposed to swim upstream (exercise, keeps their muscle tissue and organs healthy), are now crammed into tanks so tightly that they can't move, never mind swim. 2) They're medicated against the diseases that inevitably occur in these tanks. 3) They're supposed to eat plankton, but are biologically modified to eat soy and corn, both of which were also genetically modified. Your body can't sustain any of that without serious repercussions and your brain is twice as vulnerable.

"Pancreas disease (PD) is a viral disease caused by Salmonid alphavirus (SAV) that affects farmed Atlantic salmon and rainbow trout."[250]

Just like the plastic problem, farmed fish are creating disease across the oceans, it's not contained to the tanks. This is Norway: "The possible spread of viruses from salmon farms to wild fish is a major public concern. Sea trout S. trutta collected from the major farming areas along the Norwegian coast are likely to have been exposed to SAV and PRV from farms with disease outbreaks."[251]

Some fish are escaping. Literally jumping tanks and finding their way home. *Go little guys!! Swim!* "...scale reading revealed that 10% of the salmon had escaped from farms. The prevalence of PRV in wild salmon (8%) was significantly lower than in farm escapees (86%)."[252]

If 86% of the escapees (you can't help but root for them, can you?) are diseased, what do you suppose that number is for the jailbirds still in the "sustainable" tanks, and soon to be swimming in your intestinal tract, *which has holes in it from gluten.*

4) THE DOMINO EFFECT, SYNTHETIC COLORING

Whenever humans interfere with Nature, the dominos start to fall. The antibiotics being pumped into these fish are turning them gray and/or white, which is undesirable to consumers. We want our salmon to be pretty pink.

Common sense would say that if the poor fish are diseased and now turning abnormal colors, maybe this fish-farm thing is a bad idea and we should put them back in their natural habitat. Common sense? Hell no! We're human, we have better ideas... let's create even more chemicals so we can make them pink again (same chemical is used to make non-organic tomatoes darker red... since it has no natural nutrients to get its natural pigmentation).

Enter synthetic astaxanthin, made from petrochemicals, which are not approved for human consumption in several countries. Clinical trials have never been conducted on humans for this synthetic version. But since it's not being fed to humans directly, it's being fed to the fish (even though it never leaves their body), then it gets approved.

The real thing is actually good for you. Natural astaxanthin is a carotenoid from nature, and like all colorful pigments, it's a friend with benefits. The problem is, the real thing is too expensive to throw into fish tanks (and I don't know if it would survive the chemicals and medications), so they use the cheaper synthetic versions (canthaxanthin and astaxanthin).

You can't point to the real thing, talk about how healthy it is, then turn around and create an untested version from toxic petrochemicals (meant for car cranks), that we know are harmful, and claim there won't be side effects. ...Actually, I'm wrong, you can, and they are. It's in over 70% of the fish being eaten in North America already, probably higher by the time you're reading this.

And there you have it: "sustainable fish". The next generation of fish won't know how to swim, but I'm sure there's a pill for that already in the works. We're domesticating fish and then selling them as "sustainable" and "wild caught" (if the nets they're held in are in sea water, that's still "wild"). That's legal. *Your taxpayer dollars at work.* Then more taxpayer dollars for a crumbing medical system and "unexplained" illnesses.

SUMMARY

1) Toxification affects fish and seafood of all sizes and age, worldwide. Drowning in toxic chemicals and metals can still be legally organic.

2) All sea life have non-degradable (by earth and your body) micro-plastics.

3) "Sustainable fish" are genetically modified + fed GMO toxic feed + medicated.

4) "Sustainable fish" are synthetically colored with untested petrochemicals that are banned in several countries.

You obviously know I had volumes more studies, right? All I can think when I read the warnings from marine biologists is: What on earth are we doing? Why is no one listening to these scientists who are holding hard, indisputable facts?

I once had a long conversation with the founder of a fish oil company. I respectfully stated my concerns, hoping he would enlighten me with facts that I may have been unaware of. He proceeded to spend 15 minutes talking me through all the processing, filtering, extraction, and a few more steps too technical for me to remember without having pen and paper (we weren't in a professional setting, we were seated next to each other at a gala dinner).

I listened intently, and sincerely wanted to learn. I sincerely wanted good news. He finished and asked if I had questions, I had only one: "After so many steps of processing, filtering, extraction, testing, preserving, manufacturing, and packaging, what percentage of purity would you say is left in your pill, in comparison to a sardine I might have eaten 300 years ago?" ...No answer. He only reminded me our chat was off the record.

I came across another company that uses a distillation process and then another multi-step system. Okay, that's interesting, distillation could possibly get rid of metals, though metals aren't the only issue. Let's assume it gets rid of all bad stuff. But what else does it get rid of? And while all these safety steps are happening, the oil is exposed to air, and oxidizing.

The question I'm asking myself is: Why are we doing chemical somersaults and spending millions for half-adequate filtering machinery, if there are plant-based foods (that are actually higher in omega-3's than fish), that don't require any kind of manipulation. I'm all for the scenic route when it comes to driving beautiful travel destinations, but when it comes to food, I want the smartest safest shortest route from A to B.

SOLUTION: PLANT-BASED OMEGA-3's. Listed for you, with 3-minute recipes, in the Brain Food section of this book.

Thank you for reading this chapter, you're a total Champion. *Please Keep Reading...*

Common Sense

I've always been a common-sense person, abnormally so, even before I could read. 4 years old: "Dad, if water doesn't have bubbles, should those drinks with dark colors have bubbles in them? And we can't get those drinks from the side of the mountain the way we get water, so where do they come from?" *My seashell shop was doomed from the start.*

Common Sense even became something I got publicly connected to when the CEO of Health Habits introduced me as "Where Science Meets Common Sense" (thank you Doug). It stuck, and everyone started introducing me that way. My father said: *"If only they knew."*

I see life in simplistic terms. If something you're doing is hurting you, it seems to me you should stop doing it. I get genuinely confused when there are questions about things that look entirely black and white to me.

Eating a food that causes severe health issues in every country in the world, with thousands of worldwide studies and human case studies over a period of 100 years to prove it, doesn't seem a good idea. An even worse idea is to then chemically and genetically modify that food, in an attempt to force the body to process it. We're not smart enough to play with Nature like that. If we knew the human digestive system so well, 1/3 of the free world wouldn't have digestive problems.[253]

Government-commissioned gut microbiome task forces have been setting up all over the world from India[254] (specific to Celiac Disease because the problem has become a pandemic) to joint sessions being planned on the "Gut-Brain Axis" during the 40th European Congress for Nutrition and Metabolism Congress.

The main conclusion from all these PhD's is that we've only scratched the surface and barely understand the gut microbiome. That's understandable, and it's great that we're trying to learn more. In the meantime, maybe we should stop committing gut suicide by known food bombs.

There's only one solution. There aren't options. There's no point in any discussion. We don't need more studies. The Solution is: We need to start eating real food again. Pretty simple.

No science experiments, just eat real food. That means organic, for starters. Food that's grown on a farm and not in a lab, since we're not robots and not meant to be eating circuit boards. We're designed only to eat food. We're not designed any other way. Call it simplistic, but what's there to talk about?

In caveman terms: Plant seed here, add water, plant grows, gives berries. *Simple.* Put seed here, add water, flower blooms. *Simple.* Put human here, add real food, human flourishes. *Simple.*

We need food that doesn't damage anyone's gut.

Flower + poison = no bloom.

Gluten damages everyone's gut. *Everyone.* Not just people with Celiac Disease. People with CD are simply the ones reacting in a specific diagnosable way that can be labeled as a group, but everyone else is still damaging their health with gluten at some degree and in many different ways.

It's a Gluten Moment of Truth. What happens to the next generation will be determined by how much this generation understands gluten (and food in general).

PART THREE: THE SOLUTIONS

I breathe for one thing: Results. Results require Action. You were barely a year old when you started learning an entire language. Think about what's involved in learning a whole new language, and you did it as an infant. Trust me, trust yourself, you can do this...

FOOD BASICS

True Back to the Basics

Every doctor and health coach in the world is teaching people how to do things in baby steps. I'm here to advise you to skip the baby steps. You're an adult, intelligent, and powerful enough to do anything you want. If you got stranded on a desert island, you wouldn't take baby steps away from cereal boxes, you'd instantly figure it out. You'd find fruit, berries, learn how to make a harpoon, fish, forage, build a fire... you'd figure it out or you'd die.

I don't see a huge difference between fast death and slow death, do you? It's time we treated them with the same urgency.

With an instruction book, you're capable of building a house with your bare hands. Please don't allow anyone to convince you that food changes are all that hard. Don't allow anyone to take that power away from you. Your life will be different for a few weeks until you get used to things. And? If that's the toughest thing you've ever had to face in life, you've been living a pretty sheltered life. Perspective: Empathize with soldiers, physical/emotional/mental pain, sacrifices, and their families who have had to endure loss... now tell me food habits are impossible to change. Perspective.

This is about real back to basics. Not just throwing an apple into your day, but about seeing food in a new light. By the way, that's a naturally browning apple I'm referring to, not the patented one that never decomposes. True back to basics means you're asking the question: "If it doesn't brown, expire, or decompose on earth, how will it decompose in my body?"

By the way, all this focus on neuroplasticity... yes, our bodies are amazingly brilliantly resilient and can heal if given the chance. But don't rely on something that we won't understand or know how to use for another thousand years. Rely on what we know works today. If neuroplasticity was as fantastic as they're making it sound, all neurological disorders, including Alzheimer's, could be eliminated before the end of the year. *This* year. *insert buzzer here* I'm all for advancement, just avoid Magic Pill Syndrome.

You're engaged in a high stakes game, with your brain health on the line. The solution is to become a skilled player. That means you need to understand the essence of the game and not be at the mercy of the dealer or hand you're dealt. Stay with me, I've got you.

Primal people didn't need to consciously do the things we need to consciously do (and not do) to be healthy.

The myth is that they had no stress. Wrong. They had stress. The difference is theirs' was real, not chronic, and they had support. We suffer from things that didn't exist before, like Chronic Unhappiness, Exercise and Nature Deficiency (as long as the sun is still shining, we shouldn't need Vitamin D supplements, *and yet...*). There's yet another health issue emerging today that didn't exist yesterday: Social Isolation, which is making its way into the medical books as a modern health problem, creating yet more depression. So much for all this technology "connecting" people. Perhaps we miscalculated. Perhaps human contact actually requires humans instead of an electronic middle man.

And then there's the environment, the very air we breathe...

TOXIC LOAD

As of 2017, the Toxic Substances Control Act has over 80,000 toxic chemicals in its database, many of which are used commercially, which means they're in direct contact with us. These chemicals do not need to be tested for safety. Scientific American published that less than 1/5 of these chemicals are ever tested as far as how they affect human organs.[255] This stuff is just unleashed on us.

The only takeaway from this: Be aware of what you're asking of your body, control what you can so you minimize the toxic load.

PRIMAL MENTALITY

It's a mind shift to get primal, and it's helpful if you want to maintain a healthy lifestyle. I've been making primal suggestions throughout this book, this page is about consciously making a decision to live more raw and real.

Primal thinking is helpful because it becomes a filter system for you and helps you clock out marketing on your own. You ask yourself if something was possible a million years ago...

"Sustainable" medicated, genetically engineered fish from indoor tanks or even seawater contained nets... impossible in primal times. It's out.

"Dirty Dozen and Clean 15" ... impossible in primal times because everything was organic. Clean 15 is a useless ploy to placate people into not getting overwhelmed, but at the end of the day, "a little less poison" is not what anyone deserves. Out.

A spray can spewing out some non-stick chemical cocktail to scramble your eggs in (think about a caveman's reaction to that being sprayed on the stick he cooks his food on). Out.

...You see how thinking of yourself as primal helps you automatically make better decisions? No matter how clever the marketing campaign is, you'll become immune to it.

My friends have always said that when they're in doubt, they ask themselves "Would Jaqui eat this?" When you're in doubt, ask yourself:
   1) "Would this have been possible in primal times?"
   2) "Is it a modern-day necessity that I absolutely can't avoid?"
   3) "If it's unavoidable, what's the halfway point?"

...Certain supplements are a good example of that halfway point, so are water filters. Not primal, but unavoidable.

B_{12} deficiency was the reason I needed a walking stick for a few weeks. My body went into a free-fall and nutrients got stripped away within months after I had tested fine on my first blood test. Since I had tested at normal levels only 90 or so days before my body really got into trouble, we never re-tested. I don't blame the doctors on that one, because even I wouldn't have re-tested for deficiencies that soon. It's simply too unlikely, and the truth is, I was convinced I had a hidden tumor in my brain that the MRI's missed. I had a hard time imagining getting *that* sick, *that* fast, from a food trigger. Even with my primal thinking, I lost my way a while.
As soon as I found out all this was a gluten issue, I did re-test and was at dangerously low levels on certain nutrients. Just one B_{12}/Glutathione injection, and the numbness and tingling went away the next day. I haven't stopped taking sublingual B_{12} ever since, but I still overlap all supplements with food sources. No one in this lifetime will be able to convince me that man-made anything can be as powerful as a natural food source.
So that's what primal mindset is: Make as many choices as possible that are 100% primal (example: all organic, that's in your control), and do your best to be close to that with the rest. Again, no pressure. Just do your best and every once in a while, look over your shoulder: "Am I honestly doing my best? Would Jaqui walk in here and point out 5 things I can do better?"

NakedFood

If you've followed me online, you know I'm mostly raw, sometimes all raw. My company is called "NakedFood", so it's no mystery where my personal preferences are. But that's all they are, personal preferences, not what I impose on others. The mis-perception is that I'm trying to get others to become 100% raw, and that's not true. I never have. I never, once, have told anyone to go 100% raw (unless we're talking detox for a limited time period).

My message has always been: "Add more raw."

Add. More. Raw. ...To whatever diet you choose. Plant-Based? Good. Stop cooking all your vegetables all the time. Paleo? Fine. Add a raw spinach salad next to the steak. Mediterranean? Make sure dark leafy greens accompany every meal that don't involve fruit. Whatever your food choices, just add more raw. It's not that hard. And you don't need to grow a beard, stop washing your hair, and move to the jungle to eat more raw. Yes, there are some raw foodists who put out videos from the jungles of Costa Rica or wherever... don't let their stark contrast of lifestyle from yours affect your thinking. I live in a high-rise and wear heels. Add. More. Raw.

SIMPLE SOLUTION TO ADDING MORE RAW

As a bonus, I'm going to include some recipes for raw dips in this book. Why dips? Because most people don't find salads fun. But who doesn't enjoy dips? They're TV snacks, party food, and football wouldn't be the same without them. I munch on them as I write, I eat them as starters to dinner, afternoon snack... they're so rich and satisfying, they're often my main meal.

The other thing about dips is the condensation factor. How much kale would you eat in one sitting in a salad? Half a head? Maybe? But it would take two full heads of kale to make a small bowl of dip, which you could easily munch on in one sitting. I just quadrupled your intake and made it more fun.

WHY DIPS ARE BETTER THAN JUICING

1) You keep all the fiber, this is critical to health. And you won't lose elements in the process. It's not just fiber you lose when you juice, it's inevitable that you'll lose some nutrients as well.

2) Better food combining. You won't mix with sugars and fruits. You'll mix with other vegetables, good fats, and savory flavors.

3) You'll feel satiated. A juice will go right through you and then you're reaching for food half an hour later. Dips are substance food and will keep you satisfied for hours. An easy way to maintain healthy weight and not over-eat, it's still my number one go-to for weight loss. As soon as someone tells me they want to lose weight, I tell them to prepare to eat dips at lunch and dinner, chia snacks in between, with a banana/blueberry smoothie to kick off the day. Works every time. I don't know any food programs that tell you to take 500 variations of a party food and feel free to eat as much of it as you want, any hour of the day, and still be guaranteed to lose weight (and have impressive blood results). Can't argue with results.

I'm all for juicing if it's done right. But I consider juicing a supplement to a strong diet. I don't consider juicing the only healthy element in a person's life as they're trying to make up for a terrible diet, that doesn't work. It's like driving a convertible and expecting the car heater to keep you dry from the rain.

DIPS: Can't go wrong. Recipes in the next part of this section.

Organic

"Clean 15 and Dirty Dozen". My reaction to this since the first day it came out: WTF

Yes, some foods absorb chemicals more easily from the outside, but even the hardest outer shell is still growing in soil that's drowning in chemicals, getting sprayed and resprayed crop after crop. The roots of those foods are absorbing those chemicals. Forget the outside layers, the entire interior is compromised. And what's the philosophy? Eat a little less poison on the peels? *Seriously?* There are major flaws in that bad advice:

1) **GMO** (Genetically Modified Organisms) don't have to be declared by law. It's not just pesticides you need to consider, it's whether you're eating food or a biology experiment. Organic means no FrankenFood. Conventional means you're rolling the dice. The first food at the top of the Clean 15 list is corn. Over 90% of world corn is now genetically modified. Shall we go down their so-called clean list or do you already know I'll shred it to pieces? Don't make me pull out my Geek Guns and add 200 studies to this book.

2) **Cumulative Effect.** They do a study and measure the toxic load of an apple, *one* apple, but they never tell you the toxic load of 3 meals + 2 snacks + 2 beverages. That's Day 1. By Day 788 of your life (2 years and change), you're drowning in chemical overload. Liver, pancreas, thyroid... everything starts to fail. Oh, but you've been eating "Clean 15".

3) **Juicing.** Popular. If you're reading a book like this, you're probably more concerned about your health than the average person. You probably juice, or at least try to grab a green juice when it's in front of you. It takes 5 and 10 times more greens to make juice than what you could eat/chew in a sitting, that's why juices are so powerful. They're meant to be condensed nutrition, not condensed chemicals. Juice with conventional, you're now inviting the full toxic trifecta: 1) Immediate instant shock to your immune system with condensed chemicals 2) Speeding up the cumulative effect so you're toxic in a month instead of a year 3) Damaging every part of your body with genetically modified mutant food. ...And that's your "healthy green juice". Sound Advice: You're better off with no juice, it would be slower degeneration.

Conventional isn't just about pesticides anymore, it's about biological warfare hitting every unsuspecting unarmed cell in your body and brain. If you have a compromised immune system, you're taking the hit even harder than your undiagnosed neighbor.

I once had a publisher tell me they couldn't publish my work because it needed softening. "Look at this MD, he's a multiple NY Times best-seller, and he allows some flexibility, talks baby steps, these are all universally accepted approaches. If you can do the same, we love your personal story, passion, food knowledge, and would like to work with you."

No. *Hell no.* This isn't about popularity, it's about results (and integrity). People that follow me don't spend 30 years in baby steps playing hide & seek with symptoms. You deserve better. Make a decision and execute. Will it be hard at the beginning? Maybe. So what? Do you know of any major corporation that was built with baby steps and very little effort? Is your body, mind, quality of life, less important than a company producing cell phones?

When I hear "less mercury than other brands", "dirty dozen and clean 15", "GRAS" (generally regarded as safe), and every other best-selling term of their kind, my (highly-functioning and sharp) brain is screaming: What the hell are they thinking?!?!?! ...I admire their marketing skills though. You have to be talented to make an entire society accept and happily poison themselves... *this cyanide is less than that cyanide...* Seriously, impressive job on marketing. I'm nowhere as talented as these guys are and not a NY Times Bestseller. *My people just never get sick.*

Organic. Stop poisoning yourself. Make a decision, execute. Now. This moment. And hug your organic farmer. Actual hugs are great, with your buying dollars are good enough.

Know Farmers, Know Food.
No Farmers, No Food.

Food Combining

If your gut is out of balance, your brain will be out of balance. Experience has shown me that even people on their death bed won't follow food combining strictly, so here's what I'll do, I'll give you only some critical tips and not a whole chart.

TOP 2 RULES FOR BETTER FOOD COMBINING

1) Don't mix fruit with any foods except nuts and seeds. They ferment and rot in your gut and create a disaster. Eat fruit on an empty stomach, either 20 minutes before meals, or 2-3 hours after meals. (2 hours plant based, 3 hours meat).

2) Don't mix protein and carbs (yes, I know, burger and potatoes). Have veggies and carbs one day, bunless burger and veggies the next. You're still eating everything, just not at the same time. Trust me, you'll get used to it if you do it for a few weeks. And the results will be great. It's an easy no-sweat weight loss trick. ...Also notice how greens go with everything ;)

POWER TIPS

1) Before a meal, take 20 seconds and take a few deep long breaths. You don't digest food well if you're in hyper run mode. Slow your system down, even if you're driving or in public (no one will notice, do it anywhere). Just a few deep breaths can do wonders for your parasympathetic nervous system, which calms muscles in the gastrointestinal tract. It's a good habit to get into every hour on the hour, food or not. 3 Day Challenge: All waking hours, when the minute hand of the clock hits 12, you take 6 long, deep breaths. I'll bet you feel overall calmer, and food will go down better.

2) You know this, but now do it: Chew. Chew. Chew more. Do not send whole chunks of food down your system.

3) Don't drink a lot of liquids with meals, you'll dilute digestive enzymes. I drink wine, I'm not suggesting you be extreme. But this business of washing meals down with water or soft drinks has to stop (usually caused by not enough chewing or just a bad habit people do unconsciously). Either the meal needs to change or you need to start chewing. I'm shocked at the gulps of food people swallow. And please tell me you don't drink soft drinks!

4) Avocado, lemon, onion, garlic, herbs, and edible flowers mix with everything.

5) Be thankful for your food (and everything else you have that a billion people would die for). That high energy vibration will go a long way in digestion as well as overall well-being.

Juicing Correctly

Once again, I'll keep it simple and give you only 2 things to follow to maintain gut health.

1) Don't sweeten, not even with real whole fruit. You're creating fermentation in your gut by adding sugar to your juice. If you're buying pre-made juice, check the label. Does it have sweeteners or fruit? Even if they're "natural" and organic sweeteners, if there are any, skip it. There should be nothing but organic vegetables. No exceptions. I've never had it, but Candida doesn't sound like fun to me.

2) Juice only vegetables. Eat fruit whole or in smoothies, never juice fruit, and never drink fruit juice. It's simply too high a concentration of sugar, and without fiber to control it, you may as well eat a couple of candy bars. Juice only vegetables, enjoy fruit smoothies since you can't squeeze 10 pounds of fruit into one smoothie. The amount of fruit you put into a smoothie is closer to what you'd eat, so it won't be a sugar jolt. Make sense? You want the condensed nutrition of greens, you do not want the condensed sugar content of fruit, especially with the fiber gone. It's like an LSD hit to your brain when you drink fruit juice. I won't even go into what happens to the rest of your organs.

POWER TIPS

1) To make green juices more enjoyable (I took away fruit, but I'll give you something better), add ginger, lemon, cayenne (not necessarily all 3 at the same time). Ginger adds zing, lemon adds tang, cayenne/chipotle add heat/spice. That should entertain your tongue plenty and keep your mind off sugar. I once made a tomato + greens + oregano + lemon and was told: "This tastes like a Bloody Mary! I can do this!" Yes, *you can* :) 2 Week Challenge: Do cold turkey fruitless/sugarless green juices for 2 weeks, and you'll be amazed how sweetened juice will nauseate you after that.

2) Unless you have a fantastic juicer, don't waste herbs in there, you'll get barely any of their nutrients. If your juicer is centrifugal, definitely don't put herbs there (that means parsley/cilantro, not just what we traditionally think of as herbs, like rosemary or thyme). I'll post a link of the juicer (and blender) I use at JaquiKarr.com/Resources

3) Wheatgrass: The grass is gluten free, the seeds are not. Cut about half an inch from the root and cut by the 10th or 11th day of growth. If you're in a juice bar and can't ensure these criteria, choose something else if you're gluten sensitive. I never drink wheat grass at juice bars. I don't blame them, they're in business and need to consider waste, so they'll cut as close to the root as possible.

4) Squirt some lemon or lime into all your vegetable juices to slow down oxidization, both are natural preservatives. It's a good trick, but unnecessary if you're drinking your juice within 20 minutes of making it.

5) Always chew something before you drink juice. You want your salivary glands to get activated, your brain to signal your body that food is coming and to prepare digestive enzymes for it. Don't surprise your body with food that it wasn't ready for. If you're juicing yourself, simply munch on a bite or two of whatever you're juicing. If you bought your juice, keep a small container of nuts or seeds around, chew on a bite or two to activate your digestive system. Worst case scenario: Go through the chewing motions with your mouth, even if nothing is available, saliva should form, that's your sign that the go button has been pushed.

6) Storing: If you're making juice in the morning to drink later in the day:

A) Store in a stainless-steel bottle, never plastic of any kind. This will protect your juice from light and air as well as seeping plastic.

B) Add lemon or lime to preserve, you only need a squirt, it won't affect the flavor of anything you make. TIP: You can freeze tiny bits at the bottom of an ice tray so you won't need to cut a whole citrus up every time. Novelty trays for parties are great for this since they're usually in smaller sizes than standard trays.

C) Fill to the absolute brim so that air can't fit in the bottle. Top with water if you need to. Air + food = oxidization. Oxidization = getting ready to return to earth. It's the Law of Nature...

...When you get quiet for a moment and think about that last point, it makes perfect, natural sense. If food could lie around indefinitely, what kind of massive garbage dump would earth turn into? Unfortunately, our food innovations have given us the answer to that question.

Think Primal: Real food tossed away would immediately start making its way back into the earth and become fertilizer for the next crop of food (modern day terms are composting or organic fertilizing).

The point is, food was never meant to be cut up and exposed to air all that long, its very nature is telling us that. How many minutes does it take an organic apple to brown?

...But we're brilliant humans, we don't take Nature's cues, so we've invented the "Arctic® Apple". This is a genetically modified apple that doesn't brown. It's amazing how many "health" sites jumped on how great this is, "perfect for salads", which is horrible food combining, aside from the GMO side effects.

Did you know most GMO corn is not registered as food with the FDA? It's registered as a chemical. More specifically, as an insecticide called "Bt-corn" and there's a 95-page document on the FDA web site that can give you the specifics. When an apple needs a patent and a trade mark, and corn needs a patent, trademark, and 95 pages to tell me what it is, I don't classify these aliens as food anymore. "Ht-soy" is Bt-corn's cousin and next on the alien list. To avoid having aliens invade your body and brain, buy organic.

Just to be thorough, I've geeked out on the studies for GMO's (hands down, I'm the un-coolest person you know). There are hundreds showing endocrine damage, thyroid damage, male fish turning female, sexless fish, frogs growing 3 eyes, salmon instantly needing medication to survive GMO feed... it goes on and on and on. The few studies deeming GMO's safe keep pointing me to law schools. "Health and food safety: the benefits of Bt-corn"[256] published by the University of Oklahoma College of Law, in the "Food Drug Law Journal". Legal food isn't always real food.

Here's where my no-fail question serves you well. When you hear about anything like an apple that doesn't brown, stop, ask: "Was this possible a million years ago? Could I create it with bare hands on a desert island? Is it possible without machinery, labs, or synthetic chemicals?" Now put on a welder's mask and slowly step away from the radioactive apple just in case it explodes.

It's these kinds of mind shifts that'll make you see food and life *so* differently, you'll never go back to artificial living. You can imagine what goes through my mind when I see 20-year shelf life on the alien stuff they're passing off as food. Just like you don't see food when you look at a steel pipe, I don't see food when I look at 20-year shelf life on a box. Get Naked. The only real food is NakedFood.

Paleo, Mediterranean, Ketogenic

Before you read this section, please remember two things:

1) **Don't kill the messenger.** I'm giving up my peaceful idyllic surf village life to remain a Science Geek and bring you the info you don't have time to research yourself. I know all this stuff, it isn't for me. It's for you.

2) **Don't feel overwhelmed.** There's a solution to all of this. It'll require modifications from what you're used to, but it'll save your brain health. In the coming years, a new Alzheimer's case will develop every 33 seconds.[257] There's no reason for you to be one of them. Dementia because of food? You can do better than that.

One of the running themes in this book, and my entire philosophy to health, is to make up for our modern lifestyles. This isn't just about the difference between hunting for food and going online and having it delivered to your door. It's about the biological makeup of the food itself. In each example below, observe how I'm thinking and breaking things down so that you can apply the same principles to the next hottest thing that'll follow after this is published.

PALEO

During the Paleolithic Period, animal meat contained 4% fat. Animals were running for their lives (like humans were), in wild terrain, eating grass or other lean meats (like humans were), and the entire planet was organic.

Today, animals have 40-70% fat, they're sedentary, medicated, and eating things they weren't designed to eat, like grains. A cow eating corn isn't the cow we used to know (And cows weren't domesticated in Paleo times, they weren't even called cows, they were wild aurochs. We got lazy, stopped chasing wild animals, and domesticated them about the same time we domesticated grains). Salmon are being genetically modified to eat corn feed, which itself is also genetically modified. It's layers and layers of synthetic toxins and medications.

The original Paleo Diet study, going back to 1985[258] (before Dr. Cordain's marketing team commercialized and made it popular), was based on the findings of health in *actual* Paleo times, based on those lean meats and greens, and overall lifestyles. The real Paleo diet isn't based on bacon smoothies and synthetic sweeteners (though Cordain did withdraw his endorsement of artificial sweeteners in a revision after his original publishing).

Since that original 1985 study, things took a few turns, got yet more commercialized (do you remember the telephone game?) The word "modern" got used to add no-no's to the original diet, and now we have a hundred variations of Paleo, mostly promoting volumes of high-fat meat. Everyone is focusing on the juicy T-bone and forgetting that they foraged and ate mostly greens back then. The (lean) meat they did eat, wasn't every day... never mind three times a day. No one is taking any of these things into account, because...

Who would buy a diet book that suggested you walk and run hours a day, eat 90% greens, occasional fruit, and meat once or twice a week? A publisher would print about devil worshiping before they would publish that. Publishers are not non-profit organizations, they print what they think will sell.

Here's an insider piece of info: Most books are write-offs for them. They make their money on 10% of what they publish. That 10% carries the 90% that are considered financial failures. So, they need to go with the best possible odds every time they back a book. The best possible odds don't happen by printing things that no one wants to hear. The marketing team will never approve that.

The information you're getting, online, offline, on billboards, TV, radio, in smoke signals, subliminal whispers, it's highly filtered. All of it is based on either who is paying for the ad behind it, or a marketing team who has determined if the book/product/program is something the masses will buy into.

"The Paleo Diet" isn't even where it started. As the industrial age (think 200 years before WWI), brought with it illness, by 1959 we already had studies titled "Stone age diet for functional disorders"[259] ...which simply stated that it's time to get back to real food. That was 60 years ago. But "Functional Disorders" is not a sexy title... *and no shrimp wrapped in bacon...* It doesn't stand a chance against the Paleo Diet with sexy athletic bodies in its ads. Neither does "Paleolithic diet, evolution, and carcinogens"(1987).[260]

Important to note: I'm not putting the Paleo Diet down. It's a massive improvement to what most people are eating. If nothing else, it gets people off grains, dairy, and sugar. Those three alone will create a significant turnaround. It's a pretty effective diet, even when done only half-right, so there's something to be said for that (though I'd test for arterial plaque and blood thickening with that level of meat eating). But imagine what would happen if you got it totally right. Think unmodified, non-commercialized Paleo, or more specifically, food as it used to be while we were still lean nomads. That was when our health was at its best.[261] *That's NakedFood.*

MEDITERRANEAN

I was born on the Mediterranean, didn't move to Canada until I was 6, ate purely Mediterranean into my 20's before I went high raw. My parents never adopted the Canadian diet, they stayed very much Mediterranean. Except, the oceans weren't polluted then like they are now. If you skipped it, please go back and read the chapter on fish in the Brain Damage section.

There's a second element to consider: Most people aren't even aware what the actual study referring to the Mediterranean diet was about. Ancel Keys PhD, "Seven Countries Study" (1958), it was epidemiological research on a 40-year observation of several countries. It showed Crete to have the number #1 diet/health. Have you been to Crete? Have you seen the kind of rugged terrain they walk every day? I can assure you, it's not the South of France (or whatever other travel destination most people envision when they think Mediterranean) and they're not eating mashed potatoes that are 1/2 potato and 1/2 butter. *Vive la France.* Also, may I repeat: 1958. Pesticides, GMO's, and commercial food was nowhere in that study because it didn't exist yet.

The wonderful studies (based on people from generations ago) talk about how great the Mediterranean Diet is, how people in Sardinia, Greece, and other places live to be over 100 and healthy... The studies on those people's grandchildren will have very different results. Cancer, dementia, autoimmune disease, heart disease, is what you'd see if you lived long enough to see those studies. We're already seeing a rise in coronary heart disease in Greeks,[262] it won't be long before they're as bad as North America.

You can't point to a population that existed when the entire planet was 100% organic (and didn't use cars to walk their dogs) and say that you'll get those peoples' results today.

How much bitter dandelion have you eaten this week? Or ever? Not French brie, bitter dandelion. "Horta" is a Greek staple (covers all the bitter power greens: dandelion, mustard greens, chicory...). It's a massive pile of dandelion greens seasoned with salt, lemon, olive oil (And those women climb wild mountains to pick those greens, they don't drive to grocery stores with an 1100-calorie grande caramel caffè latte from the drive-thru on the way. They might have had a one-shot black espresso.) But when you see the Mediterranean Diet advertised, is it with weeds? (Dandelion leaves are the weeds that everyone sprays pesticides on to get nicer lawns). I've never seen the Med Diet with any quotes that 2-3 miles of wild, elevated, mountain walking should be included.

We ate fish almost every day when I was a kid. Sometimes on the weekend we had meat, for family feasts and celebrations (Note: Meat once or twice a week). The first time my Dad took me to a fish market in Canada, I immediately got sick, ran outside and vomited. I was nauseous all night, couldn't eat dinner, queasy the next day. ...It wasn't a question of smell, because I used to roam the fish markets with my grandfather as a kid, on the docks, as fishy as it can smell. We hopped on those boats all the time. Commercially processed, never mind medicated and genetically modified, is not the same fish as even I knew as a kid. My little newly Canadian nose knew that. We don't need to go back generations.

Once again, what publisher on earth is going to print a book talking about fish toxicity and that the Mediterranean Diet is no longer possible as we know it? No one buys bad news. ...*Thank you for being here, you're in the brilliant 1%, and your health thanks you even more than I do.*

FYI: I can easily write an 800-page book citing thousands of studies, ocean conservation groups, marine biologists, ... I included just enough to show you the state of affairs, knowing that I'm already risking you tapping out. Even the remote ends of the world are seeing complete ocean collapse and devastation, look at the title of this study: "Marine biodiversity at the end of the world: Cape Horn and Diego Ramírez islands."[263] ...*at the end of the world...* and still there's dangerous levels of toxins in those fish.

Even if we did everything right, starting this very moment, you and I would not live long enough to see the ocean return to its healthy state. In light of that, my advice: Stop eating fish. Stop eating all seafood and support conservation groups that are doing what they can to restore ocean health.

...Remember to not shoot the messenger, I'm putting myself out on the line for you. It would be easier for me to highlight that I'm Mediterranean and publish a glossy cookbook filled with beautiful photos of Mediterranean dishes, goodness knows I have enough recipes. I'm saying things you don't want to hear because I care about you and I want you to be able to remember your own name 30 years from now.

KETOGENIC

Yes, I'm aware of the short-term results. I can stake my life I probably read more than you do... *but...* but... *very big but...* I'd like to see the aging process and other side effects of the Keto people in 10-20 years. Actually, no, I'm not looking forward to seeing that.

When you take fruit out of a diet, you take away:

1) Flavonoids, which fight oxidative stress and are showing promise as a method of prevention for Parkinson's Disease, but so far studies are showing they wouldn't reverse the disease once developed.[264] That means you need to be eating fruit *before* you get sick. "Oxidative stress" is literally your cells rusting. By definition, flavonoids also have anti-aging effects. Why would you stop eating the fountain of youth?

...Before you ask, yes, vegetables and even wine contain flavonoids, but we're not that smart yet. ALL foods contain unique components. By skipping fruit and eating only vegetables, you're not guaranteed to be getting all the nutrients you need for optimal health. They all have different properties, and we've barely identified a handful of nutrients. We identified Vitamin A over a century ago. It goes alphabetically and we're still only at K.

Flavonoids "inhibit neuroinflammation [that's the death of neurons that leads to Alzheimer's and other brain disorders], increase cerebrovascular function, and improve cognitive performance."[265] We don't even completely understand how or why they work so well, we just know the brain gets a boost[266] with flavonoids. We're going to skip this brain food so we can work out less and try to fit into skinny jeans? Is that the strategy? ...Like I keep saying, humans aren't that smart... *maybe if we eat more fruit, our brains would do better ;)*

2) Antioxidants [the elements that fight off harmful free radicals that march into your system to destroy cells]. "Phosphodiesterase-9 (PDE9) is a promising target for treatment of Alzheimer's disease"[267] as well as erectile dysfunction.[268] Where do you find PDE9? In pomegranates. I won't give you the mile-high list of benefits from pomegranates, grapes, mangoes, and all the other non-Keto fruit. I'll just tell you that even a cold day in hell wouldn't stop me from eating them, I'd then be eating frozen fruit.

3) Phytochemicals, which fight and reverse oxidative stress. Phenolic compounds, a class of phytochemicals, including flavonoids and diarylheptanoids, are so powerful, they're being studied to be used as treatment for neurological disorders.[269] Brain food once again, both as a preventative measure (Parkinson's) and as damage reversal with other neurological disorders. How does it make sense to stop eating these powerhouses?

I'm good with high (good) fats, I'm *not* good with natural fruits being taken away. Fruits contain too many protective nutrients to take them away. Where would Eve be without her apple? Adam instinctively knew he should bite, *no studies needed*.

Our ancestors wouldn't have survived without the energy of fruit fueling them while they were hunting game. Since we're not as active as they were, and since we have other foods constantly available, we don't need as much fruit. But we still need fruit, for reasons we don't even know yet.

Being in a state of ketosis means burning fat. By definition, that's what keto is: burning fat. The Keto Diet is based on starving your body of all sugar and loading it up with fat, so that fat becomes the primary fuel. Your body doesn't have glucose, so it turns to stored fat for fuel, that's how Keto promises weight loss *insert alarm bell here* Your brain needs 130 grams of glucose a day to function properly. Keto is the lazy man's approach, which has neurological consequences.

Burning fat is the entire goal of Keto. You don't do that with your butt in a chair and fork and knife in your hands. You burn fat when your butt is off the chair, outside, doing what your body was designed to do. Get rid of the artificial sugar, but not Nature's power foods, which includes fruit.

Will you lose some weight off the top with Keto? Maybe. But without exercise, you won't maintain it forever, and you won't get the brain-building chemicals that exercise (and fruit) provide.

DIETS INC.

Remember the Atkins Diet? It took the world by storm. Until Atkins himself died. The death certificate said head trauma from a fall 9 days before his death (his wife refused an autopsy).

Then the Wall Street Journal got its hands on his medical files and printed about years of hypertension, heart disease, and heart attack suffered before the fall of the svelte, 258-pound e$teemed Dr. Atkin$ (where would sales be if his body, in a bathing suit, was on the covers of his books?)

A spokesperson from the medical examiner's office apologized for accidentally releasing his medical records (it was first sent to the Fleming Heart and Health Institute in Omaha, NE). I never saw an apology from the multi-million-dollar Atkins camp regarding health issues that may have resulted from people following this diet.

Ten or twenty years from now, all the Keto fallout will surface. "Oh, but we thought…". Some of these diets are coming from well-intentioned people. But most of these diets are coming from un$crupulou$ people who intimately understand that everyone's dying for a magic pill, and they have brilliant Marketing Masters who know exactly what to say to you. I've studied with both groups, I know what they're capable of, up close and personal. If you were in those brainstorming sessions, you'd be outraged at how they strategize to get your Diet Dollars.

Pay closer attention to when medical institutes talk about the Keto Diet (they have legal liability to consider). They'll usually say things like "we also suggest vigorous workouts and strength training." It reminds me of the weight loss meal replacement products that always have fine print regarding the importance of aerobic exercise for their big promises to work. You need a telescope that can see to the moon to read that ultra-fine print, but it's always there.

Do I ever recommend Keto? Sure. For short periods of time, 7-21 days, and that's if you're fighting off an illness, the same way I'd recommend supervised water fasts or juice feasts. I'm okay with it for serious illness or detox/reset from sugar, not for vanity reasons, not for shortcuts to weight loss.

Starve out sugar for a week, retrain your palate, and hit the reset button. Then get back to a healthy, well-rounded diet. The long-term damage and sad stats of eliminating fruit from the diet are something I'm not looking forward to seeing. I thought the same thing when they declared a war on fat.

BOTTOM LINE, ALL DIETS

Get yourself out of the diet game. Just pull out. I'd make a lot more money if I invented the "20 Pounds Slimmer in 10 Days Diet", but I don't do circus acts. I don't do gimmicks. I don't do catchy headlines. It's why I'm mostly offline. And it's why I get results that last a lifetime. *No panda bear on a tricycle doing circles around a ringmaster.* I'd rather see the panda in the wild, climbing trees, chewing on greens and bamboo (did you know they eat 14 hours a day in real life?)

I've been in publishing meetings where they asked me to take a renowned MD's ramblings and make his book easier to understand for the common person, then add recipes to include ingredients people loved, minimize the dreaded veggies or smother with cheese or bacon if greens must be there… (you can imagine my reaction).

Then they slap a catchy name and commercialize it with big promises. There's always a legal person in the room guiding them to word things to avoid lawsuit. ...Does any of this sound like they have your best interests at heart?

(FYI: I declined the contract that asked me to minimize greens. I've never written anything harmful, just re-written MD's medical jargon to layman's terms)

For your health and sanity, get yourself out of the kazillion dollar diet game. You're equipped with a 2-wheel tricycle and the marketing people are driving Batmobiles. Learn what real food is and it'll be the last time you ever hear the word diet.

Cheat Days

Don't do it. I know every nutritionist on earth says to have cheat days, even trainers to professional athletes say it. I used to be a trainer to athletes and you know what I used to tell them? NO cheat days.

SOLUTION TO CHEAT DAYS

Make a list of what you consider cheat food and figure out how to eat it all the time, even daily. If you're eating these foods as your regular meals, who needs to cheat? So simple, it hurts.

FRENCH FRIES: Cut potatoes, soak in water and drain (gets rid of some starch), pat dry, toss with a little coconut oil (creates exterior crunch), then bake. You can also boil the potatoes for 5-10 minutes first, it creates the perfect soft interior - this works perfectly for wedges or thick cuts. My favorite way is to bake thick wedges, then garnish Greek style: sprinkle with oregano, salt, lemon, drizzle of olive oil (try it, you'll give up ketchup forever). If you love ketchup, don't inject sugar into your body for nothing. Blender: fresh tomato, a few sun-dried tomatoes (sweetens, thickens, and also adds clean protein), tiny onion if you like, 10 second blend and you have ketchup. Splash some MCT oil in there to make it brain food. Ketchup. Brain food. *Welcome home.*

POTATO CHIPS: Thinly slice potato (ideally sweet potato and not white) with a mandolin and either bake or if you have a dehydrator, dehydrate. You can make all kinds of vegetable chips (try beet with lemon and thyme). It's usually the texture people are looking for, the crunch. All good, re-create the crunch in a healthy way and you're set. No trans fats. No hydrogenated fats that hurt your memory and retard your brain[270] (literally, "retard" meaning slow it down... which is what bad fats, especially fried, do to your entire body).

CHEESECAKE: Soak macadamia nut and cashews for a few hours, then go to my Pinterest board called "Raw Desserts" and pick from hundreds of cheesecakes with healthy crusts. I often have raw cheesecake for breakfast, with a date/flax/walnut/coconut crust (total brain food).

If I'm eating cheesecake and chocolate truffles and raw banana-blueberry ice cream for breakfast, when would I have an unhealthy craving for these things? Never, that's when, because I'm eating them all the time. You see how this works? It's never about will power. It's about satisfying all your desires with purer ingredients and clean methods of preparation.

ANY food you love that is considered a cheat food, I promise you, there's a better way to make it, and almost always even raw (not that raw is mandatory, I'm just saying it's easy to make anything in even the most ultra-healthy way). Ever tried marinated and seasoned dehydrated eggplant? *Bye-bye bacon, bye-bye brain fog, hello skinny jeans.*

TRANS-FATS (COMMON IN CHEAT FOOD) FRY YOUR BRAIN

"T-fat from the diet is incorporated into brain cell membranes and alter the ability of neurons to communicate. **This can diminish mental performance.** Relationship between **T-fat intake and depression** risk was observed. There is growing evidence for a possible role of T-fat in the **development of Alzheimer´s** disease and cognitive decline with age."[271]

You think I'm going to depress myself and contribute to Alzheimer's risks so I can eat junk food every Saturday? Why would I? I can re-create all my favorites without damaging my brain on a consistent basis. Stop committing pre-meditated brain murder.

Like I used to tell my athletes: Why would you work so hard all week, only to set yourself back for foods you can easily create in a delicious, but healthy way? It's counter-productive, harmful, and so unnecessary. I don't want to sweat for days on a treadmill just to have some junk food on Saturday. Not a chance. I have better things to do with my time than burn useless calories.

Calories aside, I also don't need to throw a wrench in my brain function for 48 hours and then work the rest of the week to detox it, only to throw toxins back in... What a useless cycle, body and brain.

No cheating. No need to. Welcome to Food Bliss. A few power tips and tricks up your sleeve, and you'll see how easy this is. Go to Pinterest.ca/JaquiKarr for thousands of free healthy recipes.

P.S. What happens when you find yourself at a party and you eat what you know is toxic? Nothing. OF COURSE I'm not talking about a Celiac or NCGS eating gluten, I'm talking about something high in sugar or over-processed, etc. NEVER cheat with gluten. But if we're talking a food that doesn't exactly fall in the pure food category, your body is more than capable of handling it. Don't feel even a moment of guilt about it. Just don't go out of your way to plan your own self-sabotage on a weekly basis.

"Enriched With"

If I've done my job right, by the end of this page, you should experience a mind shift in how you see this aspect of food. A shift that will serve you to your last healthy breath.

Here's the tip of the iceberg on "enriched with" ...

Most of North America is unaware, but there have been several health pandemics since the 1920's as a result of nutritional deficiencies. It's not just a third world problem. Iron, niacin, folate, ... I'm going to weave in and out a bit because I have several points to make, stay with me.

Folic Acid (synthetic version of vitamin B$_9$). It's called Folate when it comes from food, and deficiencies can create serious disease. There's also a very good reason the real and synthetic versions have different names.

How serious of an issue it can be: U.S. and Canadian governments mandated cereal and bread companies to enrich their products with folic acid to help control the explosion of Spina Bifida (a tragic birth defect, Google it and be prepared to be shocked). Cereal companies enriched with folic acid, and the "immediate" problem of Spina Bifida decreased. What no one measured, is the long-term effects, which I'll get to in a minute.

They've done this with many nutrients directly connected to several health pandemics related to deficiencies[272], starting with iodine in 1924. "Iodized table salt" wasn't the manufacturer's idea, nor did any consumer seek it out. That was the government recognizing a health pandemic from an iodine deficiency.

The Pellagra outbreak in the U.S. created a Niacin (B$_3$) food fortification[273] plan. Notice movies from the 1930's and 40's always have crazed people roaming the streets? Right. That was an actual outbreak of dementia, caused by a severe Niacin deficiency. Dementia is just one effect, the most famous one. Other symptoms are aggression, mental confusion, insomnia, weakness, skin issues... not fun and not minor, potentially violent.

Pellagra is a common problem in corn (maize) eating cultures worldwide and to this day[274], eating corn creates deficiencies and in turn, serious health issues, including dementia. The 4 D's of Pellagra: dermatitis, diarrhea, dementia, death. Just to be clear, that's premature death, not inevitable natural death.

We know corn creates deficiencies, we've known it for over a century. If you think issues with corn are new, no, no, no. Since the 1950's there have been studies like "CORN treatment and pellagra"[275] and "PELLAGRA and the cooking of corn."[276] In 1951, they were digging up medical papers on the issues of corn that were already 150 years old: "Indian corn and pellagra by Carlo Buccio at the Accademia bresciana in 1804 and 1805."[277] And still, corn has become one of the highest commodity foods in the world, despite what we knew long before the industry became what it is now.

Our (Canada and U.S.) governments decided to keep subsidizing the corn industry, tell consumers to eat more corn, and squirt some synthetic B_3 into those cereal boxes since they've trained every household to start their day with those boxes of foods that are incapable of expiring. *Let's not worry about the consequences, we've got this, we know everything about Nature from our 30-day lab tests on rats, and this is the solution.* ...Our taxpayer dollars at work. No real food alternates even considered.

There have been decades of concerns that food fortification "might lead to changes in epigenetic patterns... Most of the concern has surrounded cancer..."[278] and while they're still studying this, "...unmetabolized folic acid is related to cognitive impairment among seniors"[279] ...among a whole list of other potential issues I won't get into.

Solve today's problem the wrong way and you create bigger problems for tomorrow, but there's no app for that.
Now here's how twisted the whole system is: Industrial food and TV dinners moved people away from eating fresh vegetables, causing measurable, traceable, issues from Spina Bifida[280] to Alzheimer's[281]. Instead of telling the public it's important to keep eating the raw greens we've been eating for 2 million years, they tell agri-business to add a synthetic supplement, knowing there are adverse effects, and the consumer is told to eat "healthy grains", and more of them. Besides causing depression and long term cognitive decline, there's another problem with synthetically enriching wood chips, *pardon,* I mean cereal...

...Not everyone can process synthetic folic acid (which makes me wonder what underlying issues we're not aware of yet, with people who are seemingly processing it). For every synthetic food problem, there seems to be a synthetic solution loaded with side effects. I've listened to doctors discuss testing for the "MTHFR defect" [MTHFR = methylenetetrahydrofolate reductase], so if you have this "defect", you'll know you need to supplement with the "active form", etc., etc., etc.

Primal Thinking: I'd say it wasn't a "defect" but a sign of correct bodily function when my body doesn't want to process synthetic toxic stuff. It knows how to process real B$_9$ just fine.

Here's a novel idea: Eat Folate, which *no one* has a defect in absorbing. *Imagine that, we're all hard-wired to process the real thing.* 2-3 cups of raw spinach = a full day's folate. That's one salad/side dish. No adverse effects, no deficiencies, no messing around with your genes, no risks of cancer and dementia. How hard can it possibly be to eat some spinach next to dinner, or to make a little bowl of dip out of it and have it as a snack or starter before dinner?

All roads lead back to: Real organic food, *mostly green.* But don't rely on the medical system to tell you that. After everything we know, here's what they'll still be telling you for the next hundred years: "The pace of preventing these serious birth defects can be accelerated if more countries require fortification of both wheat and maize flour and if regulators set fortification levels high enough to increase a woman's daily average consumption of folic acid to 400 mcg."[282] [2009, regarding Spina Bifida].

NO mention of eating organic leafy greens.
NO mention of the epidemic health issues wheat causes.
NO mention of the indisputable nutritional deficiencies maize causes.
NO mention of synthetic folic acid linked to cancer and dementia.

That was just the school of public health. Surely, the branches of government in place to actually take care of every citizen's well-being know better, right? Ha. United States CDC: "All women capable of becoming pregnant should follow the USPHS recommendation and consume 400 microg of folic acid every day."[283] Zero warnings of anything, zero alternate suggestion of greens.

I've been at conferences with an auditorium full of PhD's and a panel of people with more education than rocket scientists, all discussing how to alter food to deal with deficiencies and health epidemics. My favorite so far: The discussion of "Golden Rice."[284] This is genetically modified rice to make up for beta-carotene deficiency. There were hours of discussion on mutations, genetic modification, genetic engineering, lab methods, you name it, most of it too geeky, even for me.

I finally put my hand up and asked the room: "What if we just told people they need to eat more carrots, peppers, sweet potatoes, mangoes, apricots, peaches… even kale and dandelion greens contain beta-carotene. That would solve the problem without causing any health risks. And all the areas where they grow rice, have the soil and climate to grow most of those fruits and vegetables. What if you guys, the elite scientists that can put together an international report that would get many governments' attention, suggested a task force to help farmers convert a few patches of soil for the nutrient rich food their people need."

…They looked at me like I had just escaped from a psyche ward (I was looking over my shoulder for security the rest of the day) and I can guarantee you, my suggestion never crossed their mind. Eat a peach? Too foreign a concept.

I'm not sure, but it's possible too many PhD's makes it impossible to think simple anymore (simple solutions also don't get you grants for studies to make your scientific mark on the world). There were a few seconds of silence after my comment, *"Thank you for your input Ms. Karr,"* and they went back to discussing best gene mutations of rice and what would pass FDA requirements under GRAS, which lab experiments killed the least rats, and how to get approval fastest. Scientists and lawyers: lethal combination.

It was a food conference and there wasn't a farmer in sight. Then again, most farms don't have farmers on site anymore either, they have engineers.

POWER TIP: The next time you see "enriched with XYZ" on a processed box, pull out your smart phone, Google "What foods contain XYZ", walk away from the box aisle, go to the fresh produce aisle and get the real thing.

RAW DIP RECIPES

How to Eat More Mushrooms, Power Tips

If you skipped it, read the NakedFood chapter, explaining why dips are a fantastic element to incorporate into your life. I'm pleased to share some of my nutritionally dense, power dip recipes with you. Alternate ingredients and you'll turn these 10 recipes into 1,000+, I've given you some variations to get you going.

Never sweeten with fruit. Never sweeten at all, train your palate to get off sugar. I know you can, *you* know you can.

Please don't eat these power dips with toxic crackers, even if they're labelled gluten free. Look for healthy crackers, chips, and breads. If you want to be a total rock star, eat them with vegetables. Bell peppers, celery, broccoli, cauliflower... all terrific for dipping and upping your vegetable intake that much more.

It's also a good way to eat other power foods raw, when you might not know how to do so otherwise. Example: Mushrooms are great for you, but outside of chopping them into a raw salad, how do you eat them raw?

RAW MUSHROOM APPETIZERS, SIDE, OR FULL MEAL

Shiitake (selenium) and White Button (B$_{12}$) Mushrooms: Take any one of the dip recipes you want and just before blending, throw in the stems of the mushrooms to the dip mix, then turn the main mushroom upside down on your plate. Make your dip (add ground flax to make it thicker), and spoon into the mushrooms. You now have sexy appetizers or snacks that feed your brain, detoxify you, and give you powerful nutrition, all at the same time.

Portobello (also called Portabella) Mushrooms: A great source of dietary fiber, contains Vitamin B$_6$, Copper, Folate, Magnesium, Manganese, Niacin, Pantothenic Acid, Phosphorus, Potassium, Riboflavin, Selenium, Thiamin, Zinc, and even Protein. It's one big piece, so even faster to make than a whole bunch of smaller mushrooms. Chop a bed of spinach, parsley, or any green on the bottom of the plate, put the gorgeous massive Portobello on it, then pile on 2 cups of any of the dips (which is more vegetable servings than most people get in a week) ... that's a meal all by itself. 10-minute prep, pure raw power, it's one of many food habits that makes me feel bionic.

With small mushrooms, I thicken my dip so the mixture will hold on them. With Portobellos, I make my dip more liquidity so the mushroom absorbs all the flavors, as do the greens I chop under it. Knife and fork situation for sure.

Construction Man Appetite Version: Chop greens on the bottom of the plate (spinach works well in this recipe), put as much cooked quinoa on it as you want, then the raw Portobello, then pour your raw dip over all of it like a thick sauce. The hot quinoa will absorb the sauce and go to a whole new level of flavor, so will the mushroom. You see how easy this is? Try that with the Sun-Dried Tomato & Red Pepper Dip, I dare you to tell me you didn't fall in love
...FYI, that would be the same protein as a steak (you wouldn't believe the protein level of sun-dried tomatoes), but a cleaner source.

EFFORTLESS AND A PLEASURE

When all these pure, rich flavors explode in your mouth, your palate will change. The synthetic weird food out of a box will become unappealing and taste strange to you (In a blind smell test, I once guessed "laundry detergent" for a salad dressing. What are the odds I'll ever find synthetic food appealing?) You'll be craving real food, with fresh real taste, all by yourself, no effort or will power needed. No will power needed means you'll maintain it.

When I used to do personal consults, people always got mystified with how I managed to get life-long results for my clients. It's because I never made them rely on will power or feel like they were deprived. I took whatever they were eating and supercharged it so much, it made their old version seem bland. Fudge squares? No problem. Have you ever had it with 100% pure real raw cacao? Sweetened with dates, so it's just as sweet as any toxic stuff, but so condensed, you can't finish a square in one sitting. It's just too rich and your body will say stop on its own.

The synthetic stuff:
1) Messes with your hard-wiring in gut and brain, disrupts satiety signals, just like a crack addict, making you want more.
2) There's zero nutrition, so your body tells you to keep eating (because it's craving nutrition and can't find any, so it pushes you for volume). Ironically, many of those foods not only are empty of nutrients, they also create deficiency, putting you on the negative side of the balance sheet (that's why people often crave food 1 minute after they had a big grain meal).

Give your body condensed nutrition and the shut-off valve kicks in. That is one of the reasons I get the results I get, and now it's in your toolbox.

By the way, that fudge square also had walnuts, Brazil nuts, macadamia, Ginkgo Biloba, Matcha, coconut oil, and flax in it. More omega-3's than three large pieces of toxic salmon, with an extra 60 nutrients that salmon doesn't have. *And that's just one small piece of dessert (or breakfast, or afternoon snack, or midnight snack...).* Welcome to NakedFood, where decadent fudge squares at 2 a.m. feed your brain and cause no guilt.

POWER TIP FOR DIPS (if you don't have a food processor): The trick with blender is to add enough water to be able to mix, then pour it into a bowl, then spoon in ground flax to thicken. You can do the same with cheesecake bases: blend dates, nuts, liquid (whether it's water or a nut milk), then spoon in flax or very finely shredded coconut and/or nut flour. So, you don't even need a food processor, though it makes it easier.

DIP: Champagne Mango & Avocado

This is my favorite recipe of all time. I don't even care about the sky-high nutrient factor, the refreshing taste is like a tropical vacation with every bite. Warning, if you make it at a party, make a gallon, *maybe two gallons,* and I still can't guarantee there won't be fist fights over the last bites.

(don't use a processor for this; mash in chunky texture with fork or potato masher)

- 1 champagne* mango (loaded with beta-carotene, which, components in the avocado make more absorbable, which makes these ingredients the perfect pair)
- 1 avocado
- 1 clove of crushed garlic
- 1 green onion (or very tiny red onion) finely chopped
- 2 tbsp flaxseed or extra virgin olive oil
- juice of 1 lime
- Pinch of salt

OPTIONAL: 1 tsp cumin powder

OPTIONAL: Sprinkle with chopped parsley or cilantro

*Tastes best with "champagne" mango, also called "Ataulfo". Wait until they're ripe (very bright yellow, a little soft to the touch). Can be made with regular mango, it just doesn't taste as explosively amazing. It doesn't taste the same at all.

DIP: Black Olive & Kale

"Dear Jaqui, this recipe is genius. I have a family of veggie-phobics. I made this dip as a TV snack and my kids finished it in 10 minutes, I actually had to do a grocery run at 9 p.m. and get more kale. I can't believe it, we went through 6 heads of kale in one evening. That's a miracle in my house."

FOOD PROCESSOR

- 3 cups kale
- 1 cup parsley
- ½ cup pitted black olives
- 4 tbsp tahini*
- 1 tbsp nutritional yeast (be sure it's GF, not all are)
- 2-3 cloves garlic
- 1 level tbsp cumin powder
- Juice of one lime (or lemon)
- 2 heaping tbsp hemp seeds or ground flax seeds

-Serve over a bed of chopped parsley
-Top with chopped tomatoes and green onions

OPTIONAL: Cayenne or Chipotle powder to taste

VARIATIONS: Substitute the kale with spinach, watercress, Swiss chard, broccoli, dandelion, rappini

TIP: An excellent habit is to use a different green each time you make it, keep it going on a rotation system

*Pure sesame butter, it's a good fat, don't be scared, I've been eating it my whole life. Happens to be a complete amino acid, which is pure protein in a very clean source. Bodybuilders: Double up quantity every time you see tahini, same for anyone healing from a surgery.

I want you to focus on flavor so I'm not weighing you down with nutrition facts (I think I maxed the Geek Talk quota throughout the book), but you should know most of these recipes are bodybuilder level of power nutrition and protein. Alternate all the recipes constantly, then see what will happen to you within weeks (Please write it in your 5-star review of this book so I can see all the success stories!)

DIP: Sun-Dried Tomato & Red Pepper

- ½ cup sun-dried tomatoes
- 1 fresh tomato
- 1 red bell pepper
- 1 level tbsp paprika
- juice of ½ a lime (or ½ lemon)
- 2 cloves garlic
- small bunch fresh basil
- MCT Oil, Extra Virgin Olive, or Flax Seed Oil to desired thickness

OPTIONAL: Fantastic additions are pine nuts, walnuts, slivers of dehydrated onion or eggplant, chives

VARIATION: Switch the fresh basil for thyme or oregano

VARIATION: Switch the red bell pepper for orange, yellow, purple. Different pigments = different nutrients. Keep it on rotation system, buy whichever looks freshest and feels firm (only green bell pepper doesn't do well as far as flavor here).

TIP: By adding tomatoes (high liquid) to this, you have an awesome salad dressing or topping for roasted vegetables or marinara sauce for zoodles (zucchini noodles). Use 3 tomatoes instead of 1 and it's a whole new game.

TIP: Using MCT oil in dips and salad dressings is high-octane fuel for your brain

DIP: 3 Bean Garlic & Lemon

- 1 cup chick peas
- ½ cup red kidney beans
- ½ cup black eyed peas
- ½ cup tahini
- 2-3 cloves garlic
- Juice of 1 lemon + some of its rind
- 3 tbsp ground flax
- 2 tsp cumin (optional)
- 1 tsp freshly ground black pepper
- 2 shallots/green onions (mix in or as garnish)
- Add water to desired texture, ½ cup works well

SERVE: In a glass bowl, layered with any chopped green. Example, chop up spinach, put a layer in the bowl, then spoon in some dip, add another layer of spinach, spoon in more dip...

LASAGNA: This dip also works fantastically for an eggplant or zucchini lasagna. Just add more ground flax to make it thicker so it'll old in place.

VARIATION: Replace the cumin powder with fresh rosemary.

DIP: White Bean & Rosemary

- 2 zucchinis
- 2 cups white navy beans (cooked or soaked* 4-5 days)
- Juice of a lemon (I like it extra tangy and add a few actual slices too, rind on)
- 8 sprigs of fresh rosemary
- ½ cup baby onion sprouts or mustard seed sprouts
- 2 tbsp nutritional yeast** (make sure it's GF)
- Pinch of salt
- Freshly cracked black pepper

VARIATION: the strong flavors of this recipe make it adapt well to eggplant in the place of zucchini

TIP: Stuff bell peppers with this an up your nutrient intake

*HOW TO SOAK: change the water a.m. and p.m. every day. You can keep the beans on your counter (glass jar of course)

**Nutritional yeast is a great source of B$_{12}$

DIP: Cauliflower Tahini

- 3 cups raw cauliflower
- 1 zucchini
- 2 cloves garlic
- 2 tsp cumin powder
- 1 tsp cayenne pepper or a small jalapeno
- 4 tbsp tahini
- ½ cup leek
- 1 tsp freshly cracked black pepper
- ½ tsp salt
- 1 oz water (adjust to desired consistency)

VARIATION: add 4 cups watercress and 1/4 cup black olives

VARIATION: If you're good with onion family, add more leek

DIP: Red Pepper & Greens

- 1 red bell pepper
- 3 cups kale
- 5 cups watercress (or spinach)
- 2 cloves garlic
- juice of 1 lime
- 1 cup dulse (sea vegetable)
- 2 tsps cumin powder (optional)
- 1 tsp cayenne pepper
- ½ cup tahini
- 1 cup chick peas
- 4 tbsp ground flaxseed
- 1 cup black olives
- ½ cup water
- ½ cup chopped walnuts

VARIATION: Add a raw beet

VARIATION: Replace walnuts with pine nuts, both can also be omitted, won't affect flavor

DIP: Watercress & Leek

- 3 cups watercress
- 1 cup leek (try to get both green & white parts in, double up the entire recipe if needed)
- 1 cup spinach
- ½ cup tahini
- juice of ½ lemon (or 1 lime)
- 2 tsp cumin powder
- 2 cloves garlic
- 1 hot* pepper of any variety, jalapeño works fine too (omit completely for mild version)

VARIATION: Top with a cup of chopped vine-ripened tomatoes for extra fresh taste, or grated carrots for sweetness since we're using bitter greens. ...That's a really good trick for all these recipes for you bitter-green newbies: add carrots for sweetness.

VARIATION: Replace watercress with dandelion or rappini

*TIP: Omit all hot spices if you are in damage control mode

PESTO: Garlic & Parsley

- 3-5 cloves garlic (alright, not the most date-friendly, but if you both eat it, you're fine ;)
- 3 cups parsley
- Juice of 1 lemon
- ½ tsp salt
- MCT, flax seed, or olive oil to desired consistency
- ½ cup walnuts

VARIATION: Replace parsley with any herb. I love basil and thyme for this. Basil is always my favorite pesto green.

VARIATION: Replace walnuts with pine nuts or pistachios

TIP:
Basil, stems included
Thyme, leaves only, stems are bitter

HUMMUS (which are all dips): Red Pepper

- 1 red bell pepper
- 2 cups chick peas
- Juice of 1 lime (or ½ lemon)
- 1 tsp freshly cracked black pepper
- ½ cup tahini (optional)
- ½ cup sun-dried tomato or 1 small tomato (or both)
- 2 tbsp ground flax (add 1-2 more if using fresh tomato)

VARIATION: ½ cup black olives and thyme

VARIATION: Replace the chick peas with white navy beans

VARIATION: Replace red pepper with yellow, orange, purple

BRAIN FOOD

Food List

DON'T BE AFRAID OF GOOD FATS
The boundary between brain cells is fat, never be afraid of good fats. I eat tons of avocado and tahini, their fat content is total brain food. Not just the brain directly, but all the cells, neurons, molecules *insert list of brain components here, which I'm convinced we barely know yet* that help your brain work, as well as communicate to the rest of your body. Good fat (raw natural food) is great, bad fat (artificial, processed, fried) is destructive.

EAT ALL FRUITS AND VEGETABLES
There are superstars like broccoli that we know of, but you know where I stand on this: We're not smart enough to have this all figured out, so eat all fruits and vegetables you can find in organic. I suggest "eat all greens" (including the ones you've never tried before), but I can hear your question across the miles: "Which are the most powerful?" Alright, you twisted my arm...

Power Greens: Broccoli and Broccoli Sprouts, Parsley, Kale, Watercress, Dandelion, Coriander (Cilantro), Swiss Chard, Brussel Sprouts, Mustard Greens, Spinach, Collards. *(I was cringing writing that... I seriously suggest you eat everything from the plant kingdom you can find in organic)*

POWER TIP: Double up on your greens by lining or bedding.

"Bedding" in the NakedFood kitchen means chopping up any green and putting it on your plate before anything else. That creates your bed, now put on whatever it is you were going to eat. Be patient and experiment until you figure out which flavors enhance your meals best. The sweetness of dill or coriander is perfect to bed under eggplant. The bitterness of dandelion or watercress stand well under the sweetness of red bell peppers or sweet potatoes. You see how you balance flavors? Sweet + Bitter = Balance.

"Lining" means a layer of greens you'll never even notice. Collards are awesome for wraps or to make maki rolls. Lay down the collard, now line it with spinach leaves, then add your fill and roll. You just got a layer of spinach you hadn't planned to eat. For maki rolls, insert toothpicks (I use a metal re-usable set) and cut your rolls... they now look like fancy appetizers, it's pleasing to the eye and easy to eat, you just pick up each toothpick. Line your GF bread/sandwiches/wraps with greens, including herbs and sprouts. You'll never know they're there, your body and brain will.

KETO PEOPLE: I know you're squirming at the thought of eating fruit and were convinced you were on to the right thing. If you skipped that chapter, go back and read "Paleo, Mediterranean, Keto". And you should know that flavonoids (one of many power components of fruit) are being looked at as therapy to heal the gut specific to neurological disorders, or as they call it in the study: "Neuropsychiatric Disorders."[285]

If you still feel absolute reluctance (I've been in health for decades, I know exactly what and why you're feeling it, and it's totally cool, everything in its time), at a minimum, get blueberries and raspberries on your list of staple foods.

FYI All: Note the beginning of the title of that study: "Gut-Microbiota-Brain Axis and Its Effect on Neuropsychiatric Disorders...". That axis they're referring to, your whole body is obviously connected, but there's a solid triangle between your gut, brain, and mood. It's not just about keeping criminals out of your gut, it's also about populating it with natural-law-abiding citizens, so that The Republic of You is a good place to live.

STAPLE FOODS, BESIDES ALL VEGETABLES AND FRUIT

-Avocado (both fruit and veg, but deserves special mention)
-Brazil Nuts (for selenium)
-Blueberries (and all berries)
-Chia Seeds
-Dried Apricots (clean source of iron, easy to carry around)
-Flax seed oil and ground flax (never heat the oil, use in smoothies, sauces, dips, salad dressings, or as drizzle on food)
-Kombucha*
-Matcha Green Tea (1 cup Matcha = 10x EGCG of regular green tea)
-MCT oil (8 or 10) or spoon of coconut oil daily (make it a ritual)
-Raw Cacao** (complex antioxidants and great for magnesium)
-Sauerkraut (natural probiotics, take a few bites before lunch or dinner)
-Sea Vegetables / Blue Green Algae (make it a staple if you're all plant-based, this one tip will help avoid issues)
-Tahini (clean complete amino acid and so much more)
-Turmeric
-Walnuts (omega-3's)

*Kombucha** is probiotic rich fermented tea that fizzes like champagne. You can make gallons at home for just a few dollars, it's a very inexpensive alternative to probiotic supplements.

Cacao / chocolate can be a cross-reactor with Celiac Disease, avoid if symptoms occur. Stay off it 6 months then try again, some cross reactions go away as your system gets stronger, but give it a decent amount of time (6-12 months).

Turmeric, Why and How

I say inflammation, and you think what? Most people think mosquito bite equivalent: *You eat something, maybe get a little inflamed, and you're fine the next day...*

"...gastrointestinal inflammation is a relevant pathology in schizophrenia"[286]

...No mention of CD or NCGS, this is just an out of balance, inflamed gut, which can create neurological issues in anyone. As a society, we're drowning in inflammatory diseases, and gluten is one of the worst culprits. Turmeric is the #1 anti-inflammatory in the world, for 5000+ years that we know of. That puts it on the NakedFood staple list.

Even modern medicine is catching up to ancient wisdom and acknowledging turmeric as a treatment for depression[287] and other neuropsychiatric issues from mild right up to PTSD[288]. It's shown results as both a preventative component (cancer) and treatment to many non-neuro disorders[289]. Australia thinks it can slow down progression of Alzheimer's[290], they're investigating how to maximize use.

I strongly suggest getting turmeric in your diet as often as you can, which can be daily if you get a few aces up your sleeve. Consider me your new dealer and I don't want Vegas to win ;) You know the why, here's the how...

1) WARM OR ICED LATTÉ

This alone gives you a regular dose if you make a coconut milk latté a habit the way we do with coffee or tea. Any plant-based milk will do, I suggest coconut simply because it's a little sweet and will offset the bitterness of the turmeric, hopefully preventing you from sweetening. If you do, do it with a bit of honey or maple syrup, avoid all other sweeteners. If you have the time and access to a blender, you can also blend a few dates with water or milk, warm it up, and you're set.

POWER TIP TO SWEETEN ANYTHING: A good trick to sweeten anything naturally... Blend dates with water and you have a safe liquid sweetener. How easy is that?

POWER TIP FOR DAILY LATTÉ: Alternate between turmeric and Matcha Tea powder, rest of the recipe stays the same.

2) SOUPS AND SAUCES

You can add turmeric to almost any soup, sauce, dressing, without noticing the flavor change. And it holds up nutritionally to heat, so it's great to cook with.

5 Second Soup Recipe: Cauliflower, coconut milk, turmeric = awesome soup. 5 second recipe, 30 second prep. Garnish with a heaping cup or two of chopped dill, parsley, or cilantro to add a fresh green boost.

TIP: Stop thinking of garnish as a sprig of parsley and make it a large handful. We're under-utilizing the opportunity to top our foods with green power.

Easy Drizzle Sauce (can be stored): Flax seed oil (in a dark jar, to protect it from light), add lots of turmeric, then optional ingredients like cayenne pepper, black pepper, bay leaf... shake it up, keep it in the fridge. Now drizzle on anything and everything you eat. TIP: I use the first 1/3 of my flax oil for salad dressings, then I add turmeric right to that bottle and it becomes spicy drizzle for hot soups, gazpacho, salad, quinoa, roasted vegetables, almost anything.

POWER TIP: In savory foods like salad dressings, I find I can offset the taste with cayenne or chipotle powder. Makes no sense, hot with hot, you'd think you need something sweet, but it actually works. I love that rich color too, it's beautiful when mixed with flaxseed oil then drizzled all over cauliflower soup or cauliflower mash. Chop fresh cilantro and green onions on it and wow.

3) EXPLORE. You'd be surprised at the things you can mix turmeric into. I have a client who mixes it into scrambled eggs and omelets. Her kids and husband never know the difference. Mix it right into the mustard jar, it'll add kick and blend in invisibly. Outside of vanilla ice cream or macadamia and white chocolate truffles, turmeric can go onto a lot of foods easily.

POWER TIP: "JAR #3" Do you see how easy it is to supercharge your body without *that* much effort? It seems colossal to people sometimes, just because they're not used to it. Hey, you know how to sprinkle salt and pepper on your food, right? Alright, just add a third jar to the table and start sprinkling turmeric. Keep it in plain sight so you get used to its presence, just like salt. If you tend to eat at your desk at work or grab lunch from the cafeteria, keep a small jar of turmeric in your desk and sprinkle some on. It's not colossal effort, just colossally great results.

Blueberry Brain Fuel Smoothie

BLUEBERRIES are one of the most powerful foods in the world, literally brain food, fantastic for improving memory[291] and cognitive function[292]. They're also great for improving mood[293].

The benefits don't stop there. Packed with powerful antioxidants, vitamins A, B's, C, E, iron, selenium, and zinc – blueberries neutralize free radicals thereby reducing risks to cancer[294] (particular compound in them called pterostilbene), heart disease, and have neuro-protective effects[295]. They also promote healthy urinary tracts, help prevent macular degeneration and cataracts, and even help with digestive issues. One of the richest sources of antioxidants in the world and low on the glycemic index. You definitely want to eat as many blueberries as you can.

POWER TIP: Wild blueberries are best because they have to fight tougher elements, so they develop that much more powerful components. I keep two large bags of organic wild blueberries in my freezer at all times.

BRAIN FUEL SMOOTHIE RECIPE

- 2 cups blueberries (fresh or frozen)
- Pinch of cinnamon (blood sugar balance)
- Shot of MCT oil (brain and body fuel)
- Eye dropper of liquid trace minerals
- 1 tsp Ginkgo Biloba
- Coconut Water is king for electrolytes, or water, nut milk, or coconut milk

OPTIONAL: banana (nutrients, energy, creamier texture)
OPTIONAL: ½ tsp Matcha powder
POWER TIP: Alternate Ginkgo Biloba with Siberian Ginseng every other time you make it.
...Anything goes. If you're supplementing for a specific deficiency, this is a good place to put it.

POWER TIP: Swirl every sip of smoothie under your tongue as long as you can before swallowing. You'll absorb nutrients via salivary glands and your brain will get an advance signal that the food of Gods and Goddesses is coming.

P.S. Want more smoothie recipes? "108 Smoothie Recipes with Scientifically Proven Power Ingredients + Nutrition Tips" Details at JaquiKarr.com/Books

3 CLEAN PLANT-BASED SOURCES FOR OMEGA-3s
(values are all based on 100g)

1) **Flax Seed Oil** (53,304mg of omega-3, compared to 35,311 from fish oil. Salmon is the highest source of omega-3's in the fish world, and it's still significantly inferior to flax.)

2) **Chia Seeds** (17,500mg)

3) **Walnuts** (9,000mg)

HOW TO GET MORE PLANT-BASED OMEGA-3s

FLAX: The easiest way is to use flax seed oil as your salad dressing or drizzle (never heat). 100g (7 tablespoons) of flax seeds themselves have a little over 22,000mg. Start using raw ground flax to make raw energy balls, chocolate truffles, raw desserts... Get used to sprinkling it everywhere you can, you'll never even know it's there. TIP: You want the ground version. The full seeds themselves are too small for your teeth to properly grind down, you end up not absorbing full power.

CHIA: See the next chapter for a 1-minute solution, with a thousand recipe varieties. It makes a perfect, easy, filling, nutritious breakfast. Put them in small mason jars, you can take them to work. They're filling, and excellent whenever you get hungry (say goodbye to 3 p.m. vending machine sins).

WALNUTS: Ultra-easy snack to carry around, munch on them raw (while everyone else reaches for toxic pastries and donuts in meetings). Walnuts are also great in green pesto, raw desserts, energy bars, ...

There are hundreds of ways to use flax oil, ground flax, chia, and walnuts. All this panic about omega-3's and people putting their health at further risk with toxic metals, chemicals, micro-plastics... and I can't find enough time in the world to experiment with the hundreds of luscious recipes I want to keep creating with just these 3 foods alone.

Chia Pudding

THE SIMPLE BASE (which can be all you eat if you choose): Soak 1 part chia to 2 parts water, then add any flavor you want. That's it. 10 second recipe.

How long you soak depends on the brand, some are ready in 10 minutes, others need an hour. You make a big batch, and there's your powerful omega-3 breakfast or snack for the entire week.

To speed things up or to enjoy warm, mix chia with hot water and it's ready in a minute. Just be careful: Some brands have probiotics in them, never add heat to that, you'll kill the probiotics.

FLAVORS AND FOODS TO ADD

-Raw Cacao Powder
-Cinnamon (boil a stick like tea, cool, and soak in that water)
-Nuts and seeds
-Nut Butters
-Dried Fruit
-Shredded coconut (adds flavor, texture, and natural fiber)
-Spices like nutmeg and cardamom
-Orange blossom or rose water
-Vanilla (best if you can scrape the pod of real vanilla, then throw the pod itself into your mix to keep soaking)
-Açaí (superfood, tastes like berries, beautiful rich color). There are a lot of superfoods that will add strength, taste, and color to the mix. I recently got a dried blueberry powder, try Maqui, Baobob, Matcha, Moringa, Maca... they add antioxidants and each have unique nutrients of their own.

POWER TIP for MEMORY AND FOCUS: Add Siberian Ginseng or Ginkgo Biloba (I alternate each batch), you'll never even know they're there.

POWER TIP for DEPRESSION (though this is good advice for everyone, we could all use brain boosts, I call this The Enhanced Base Recipe): Layer on the various omega-3's. You have your base of chia + water, now add a heaping tablespoon of raw walnut butter so you add omega-3's and get a creamier texture. Then add a spoon of ground flax seed. That 3x mix could be your base pudding recipe. Talk about the right way to start your day or get a lift anytime.

All of the above can be added when you make your big batch. One simple little cup of food and look at everything in there! There's more...

ON-THE-SPOT TREATS
Have your chia base soaked and ready, then add...

1) APPLE PIE
Blend a whole apple (cut the core out but keep the peel, organic of course), then mix into chia (don't put the chia pudding in your blender, it gets sticky and is hard to clean). Add cinnamon, walnuts. You increase the omega-3 content with the walnuts, and it tastes like apple pie. You shouldn't need to sweeten, but: a bit of maple syrup is okay.

2) ORANGE & GINGER
Blend a whole orange (use some of the peel, get all the pith in, that's the white part, it contains fiber and as much Vitamin C as the fruit itself), with a small piece of fresh ginger. Add chia pudding and cardamom. Done. Optional: sprinkle with raw cacao powder.

3) CHOCOLATE
Chia, 1 spoon of raw cacao per portion, hazelnuts do great here. You might also try soaking the chia in coconut milk instead of water or add shredded coconut to the mix. If you sweeten with banana, eat immediately. If not, you can store for over a week.

4) BANANA CREAM
Blend or smash a ripe banana with fork (that's sweet, you definitely shouldn't need to sweeten if you're starting with banana). Add chia pudding, nutmeg, pecans (or any nuts, but I find pecans are terrific here).

5) TROPICAL
Banana, chia, shredded coconuts, and pineapple chunks. I served this once at an afternoon tea and my friend said: "I thought you were anti-sugar, this can't possibly be so good all naturally."

You see how easy this is? Including time to wash the blender, it's under 3 minutes, and you don't even need the blender for all of them. ...Now tell me how it makes sense to expose oneself to the toxins of fish oil, when you can have omega-3's through clean plant sources in luscious desserts.

Remember, don't prep ahead with fresh fruit, they'll oxidize. With fresh fruit, don't delay eating longer than the time it takes to drive to work (if the plan is to eat at your desk). Ideally, you always eat fruit immediately after cutting. Also, as far as food combining, never combine fruit with anything but nuts and seeds (chia is a seed).

175

If you don't have time for raw fruits, that's fine. You can use cacao powder for chocolate (add nuts if you like), or Açaí / Maqui / Berry Powders to get a berry flavor (seeds go great here). Both can be pre-mixed an entire week ahead.

If you have extra-rushed mornings, I suggest you make your batch on the weekend, you can split the batch if you want a variety of flavors through the week, then spoon into small mason jars. In the morning, you grab a mason jar and go. There's your power breakfast or afternoon snack with zero time needed.

Not only are you starting your day off with brain food, but it's filling, and it feels like you're indulging in dessert.

POWER TIP: Add a few organic Brazil nuts to all of the above and you'll have a full day's worth of selenium.

Q: "What if I don't have the 10 minutes to prep this on the weekend?"
A: "It's time to re-evaluate your entire life and priorities if you can't find 10 out of 10,080 minutes a week for brain health."

Water

Seems insane that I need to write about water, but then again, the fact that this entire book (or my profession) are necessary seems insane to me every single day.

Given 60% of the human body is made up of water, you'd think there would be exhaustive studies on what happens with dehydration. We're practically relying on a 1945 study[296] that broke it down organ by organ (73% of your brain is water). There have been other studies, a little more modern...

"When dehydration reduces body mass by more than 2%, it has been consistently reported that mood is influenced, fatigue is greater, and alertness is lower... cognition of children improved in response to water consumption."[297]

There are a lot of bits and pieces, like cognitive function being lower with dehydration in younger subjects as well as elderly.[298]

I'm not the only one thinking we've ignored a critical part of health, one dude named a whole study: "Water: an essential but overlooked nutrient."[299]

We don't need science to tell us that no part of our body can possibly be functioning optimally if it's starved for water. And I'm going to pretend I'm a telepath for a second and assume you agree.

Not only do your body and brain need plenty of clean water to function properly, they need to be protected from toxic water so they don't malfunction.

CLEANER WATER

1) Avoid plastic bottles. Nothing more should need to be said here. Please don't make me pull out a pile of studies. And before you say "but I'm careful, I buy only bottles that are BPA-free" ... right, and how do you suppose manufacturers create the same flexibility they needed once they removed the cancer-causing BPA? Change the formula, call it BSA, get a new patent, run with that for a few decades until enough studies link it to cancer too... remove BSA, start again, the alphabet is useful that way.

Get yourself out of the revolving door that only leads back to illness, the house always wins in that game. The law is on their side. The only thing you can do is take yourself out of the mix. No plastic, I don't care how it's labeled. It's bad enough some plastics are unavoidable (I haven't cracked the code on how to get and store frozen blueberries without plastic).

2) Filter (option A). Reverse Osmosis will strip water of all harmful toxins, but it will also strip it of its minerals. If you go this route, get liquid trace minerals and add it to your drinking water. Ideally you put a filter system throughout your house so that you're showering (skin breathes and absorbs) and brushing your teeth (first line of absorption is your saliva, don't start and end your day with toxins) with clean water.

3) Filter (option B). High quality filter for drinking/cooking water, obviously easier than a reverse osmosis system throughout the house. The one I recommend is as powerful as what hospitals use for kidney dialysis. Can't get better than that. Link at JaquiKarr.com/Resources ...They also have a portable bottle that's affordable (stainless steel product called "pHandOrp", not the plastic one), so you can take it anywhere and have clean water.

Suggested Documentaries:
"Flow: For Love of Water" is sobering on the health element.
"Blue Gold: World Water Wars" is alarming on many fronts.

Control what you can, don't stress on what you can't, it's easy to get caught up in insanity. But being aware is good.

DEFICIENCY CREATES DEVASTATION

"Notably, essential vitamins, minerals, and omega-3 fatty acids... are exceptionally deficient in patients suffering from mental disorders... Supplements that contain amino acids also reduce symptoms, because they are converted to neurotransmitters that alleviate depression and other mental disorders. Based on emerging scientific evidence, this form of nutritional supplement treatment may be appropriate for controlling major depression, bipolar disorder, schizophrenia and anxiety disorders, eating disorders, attention deficit disorder/attention deficit hyperactivity disorder (ADD/ADHD), addiction, and autism."[300]

SPECIFIC TO ALZHEIMER'S

"The current data show that patients with Alzheimer's disease have lower [brain/cerebrospinal fluid] CSF/brain availability of DHA, choline, vitamin B_{12}, folate, vitamin C, and vitamin E."[301]

Supplement List

Do you need all these? Definitely not. A lot depends on your diet and how much damage control you have to do. For me, within those short months of initial testing until after diagnoses, I had tanked abnormally fast. Not just supplements, I took injections and I.V. treatment. B_{12} and Glutathione injections instantly, then an enhanced Meyer's Cocktail I.V. a few times.

Test for deficiency if possible. Ideally at the start of a new diet makeover, and then once a year, or every other year, to monitor where you are. You don't need to be obsessive about it. The good and bad news about most disease is they're degenerative, so they take time. As long as you monitor every other year or so, you can get ahead of things. Test for antibodies, not just nutrient deficiency.

TIP: This list doubles as a checklist for tests and note that almost none of these are tested in annual check-ups. I have no idea what they accomplish in those standard check-ups, I never bother. Even when they test for cholesterol, over 50% of people who have heart attacks had been in the normal range, so some screws need to be tightened before I'm on board. Take control of your health and ask for the things you want tested. *Your* body, *your* health.

A FEW THINGS TO NOTE AS YOU REVIEW THE LIST

1) Notice how many things sea vegetables are great for. It's amazing how powerful they are that they can rid themselves of the toxins in the ocean (something fish can't do) and then help your body rid itself of toxins while nourishing it at the same time. Hopefully, that won't change as we keep worsening ocean health. As of this publishing, sea vegetables are still a staple for me.

2) I'm providing plant-based options because these will be more bio-available for everyone. It's not meant to suggest your personal food choices, those are personal.

3) Notice that several ingredients repeat, so by having them as staples, you cross off several nutrients at the same time. Embrace broccoli :)

Don't get overwhelmed, you don't need all this. I've even indicated which ones I suggest to not use supplements for, but you should know what they are and consciously put their food sources on your plate regularly.

DO NOT: look at the list and think OMG. I don't have the luxury of giving you a personal consult and narrowing it down for you, so I'm giving you full list and the guidance you need to narrow it down yourself.

DO: Read slowly, see which ones apply to your life, highlight them, and you'll be left with a manageable handful.

Listed alphabetically, not in order of importance [food sources next to several of them]

-Alpha Lipoic Acid Your body produces it, and it's in foods you can easily eat every day, you should not need to supplement. It's a fatty acid that's in every cell of your body and here's why it's on this list: It fights the free radicals attacking your brain. They're looking at ALA as treatment for Alzheimer's[302], so it's got my attention. [Broccoli, Spinach, Brussel Sprouts, Tomatoes, Peas]

-B$_{12}$ The WGA in wheat blocks the intrinsic factor protein[303] (needed for how B$_{12}$ is mostly absorbed). If you're newly diagnosed, chances are you have some gut healing to do, so bypass the gut and supplement sublingually to ensure absorption. I recommend this for everyone, CD or not, suspected damage or not, sublingual simply provides better absorption of any vitamin.

B$_{12}$**TIP:** Look for methylcobalamin. Avoid **cyan**ocobalamin (the "cyan" is from it being cyanide based, cheaper way to make it... *don't get me going*).

"It is possible that some of the decline in cognitive function associated with aging is preventable or reversible with improved vitamin nutriture, especially vitamin B$_{12}$, vitamin B$_6$, and folate."[304]

-B Complex (check if B_{12} is included so you won't need to supplement B_{12} separately) Hard to list foods, I'd need a separate chapter since each B will have a list of its own. Nuts and spinach are up there. Online, you'll see mostly meat/egg/liver. If you're eating a lot of vegetables and occasionally some nuts and seeds, you shouldn't need to supplement. I personally don't take a B-Complex, I only take B_{12}.

-Bioflavonoids You shouldn't need to supplement [Citrus, Peaches, Nectarines, Strawberries, Grapes, Apples, Cranberries, Blackberries...] And yes, it's in wine, but what they don't tell you is you need to drink 150 glasses to get any benefit. *Poor liver.* I'm a wine drinker, I'm not saying stop drinking, I'm just saying get your nutrients and antioxidants from fresh grapes and other fruits and veggies, not alcohol (100 more points for the Marketing Masters. They did a good job, the entire world bought into it. But it's easy to sell what everyone wants to hear.)

-Biotin Marketing promotes it for nice hair, but deficiency can actually cause neurological[305] issues, *it's just not as sexy to promote.* You shouldn't need to buy supplements here, it's in a lot of foods. [Almonds, Walnuts, Sunflower Seeds, Green Peas, Lentils, Cauliflower, Avocado, Raspberries]

-Carnitine Listed because it's essential to brain health, but your body makes carnitine if you're getting all your amino acids, I don't suggest supplementing, just make sure you're getting all your essential amino acids (one of the reasons I use tahini often). [Avocado, Asparagus]

-Chromium Again, you shouldn't need to supplement. [Brewer's Yeast, Broccoli, Sweet Potato, Raw Onion, Green Beans]

-CoQ10 I suggest supplement + food. Boosts mitochondria (power generators of your cells, healthy mitochondria are critical to brain health), happens to be great for anti-aging, plus more. [Spinach, Parsley, Broccoli, Cauliflower, Avocado, Sweet Potato, Blackcurrants, Strawberries, Apples, Grapefruit, Pistachios, Walnuts, Hazelnuts, Sesame Seed (tahini), Olive Oil]

The Department of Biochemistry, Amala Institute of Medical Sciences, India, is suggesting 'Mitochondrial Medicine' as treatment for dementia (if in early stages): "A mild to moderate improvement in dementia is possible with therapy using antioxidants viz coenzyme Q10 (ubiquinone), α-lipoic acid, selenium, omega-3 fatty acids and vitamin E."[306]

Folate / Folic Acid A critical nutrient. If you skipped the "Enriched With" chapter, go back and read it. You shouldn't need to supplement, but you definitely should be getting a lot of folate.

-**Ginkgo Biloba** Easy to add to smoothies or energy bars, my desserts are laced with them :) Also add to chia mix, which I need to rename to brain mix. I see Ginkgo Biloba more as a food ingredient (like turmeric) than a supplement.

> "Furthermore the daily intake of ginkgo biloba extract can enhance cognitive performance and has been proved to delay cognitive decline in dementia. A proper dietary composition with regard to the ratio of carbohydrates to proteins, as well as the inclusion of sufficient micronutrients, seems to be favourable in the maintenance of cognitive function in the elderly."[307]

-**Glutamine/Glutamate** Glutamine helps function in your gut, brain, and immune system. Glutamate helps your cells talk to each other. The average person should not need to supplement, it's in foods you can eat daily. Exceptions: PTSD, ASD (Acute Stress Disorder), or high trauma, glutamate/glutamine may be helpful.[308] [Beets, Cabbage, Spinach, Carrots, Parsley, Brussel Sprouts]

-**Glutathione** is a molecule that not only protects your cells from oxidative stress, it also detoxifies your body. Can help get mercury out of the brain, so this is a big one. I suggest it for 2 years if you're coming off a fish diet (detoxing the brain is a slow process). Neuroscience Research Australia has measured lower levels of glutathione in Alzheimer's and MS patients, as well as those suffering from depression and other neuro issues[309]. Even with my stellar food choices, I double up and supplement, I think this one is worth it. [Broccoli Sprouts, Cauliflower, Kale, Collards, Cabbage, Brussel Sprouts, Garlic, Parsley, Spinach, Beets].

-**Iron** [Seaweed, Dried Apricots, Sesame/Tahini] I don't suggest supplementing unless you have measured low in a blood test. Too much iron isn't as harmless as too much water-soluble vitamins. I like accuracy all the way around, water-soluble or not.

-**Magnesium** Most people are deficient. Magnesium tends to drop when we're stressed, and who isn't stressed? Can solve insomnia issues in days if it's the culprit. [Dark Leafy Greens, Seaweed, Raw Cacao]

-MCT Oil (look for 8 or 10) Brain food, end of story. Good ones are expensive (and worth it). I chug it right out of the bottle. Less expensive, though not as condensed: Put a spoon of raw, cold-pressed, organic coconut oil under your tongue every day and let it melt slowly. In both cases, opt for highest quality versus quantity (which is how I feel about all foods and supplements).

-NAC (N-acetylcysteine) Can help you make more glutathione. Plenty of foods contain it, you shouldn't need to supplement unless you have something clinical going on and a professional health care provider suggests it. [Broccoli Sprouts, Collards, Kale, Cabbage, Kohlrabi, Mustard Greens, Rutabaga, Turnips, Bok Choy, Chinese Cabbage, Arugula, Horseradish, Radish, Wasabi, Watercress]

-Omega-3 [Flax Seed Oil, Chia, Walnuts] If you're suffering from clinical depression, you probably need more than you can eat in foods until you get to homeostasis. Look for a high quality DHA, preferably plant source, or at least certified to be chemical free. Don't worry about the EPA ratio, it's the DHA you want to max on. DHA has shown to improve depression[310] and neuro issues in children[311] too (autism and ADHD kids measure low on DHA). Doses vary. The standard is 1,000mg/day. I've seen papers of doctors treating severe depression with 4,000 and 5,000mg/day. Keep in mind that natural methods take time, so don't expect to be feeling better instantly, give it several months. ...That means you're committing to a somewhat expensive experiment.

SIDE NOTE: DHA / Depression. My experience with depression is that there's usually a lot of different things going on. While DHA might be helpful, I usually don't see it solving the issue by itself. Find a qualified practitioner who has experience with both clinical levels of detox and clinical levels of strengthening the system. You need a comprehensive action plan to slay that dragon, and it needs to take your specific situation into account. TIP: A good practitioner will ask you for most recent blood work and nutrient deficiency results. Get that run before your first consult and it'll save you one consult fee.

-Prebiotics and Probiotics (see next chapter)

-Selenium Critical supplement for the thyroid [Brazil Nuts: 5-7 nuts are a full day's worth, so you should never need supplements. Shiitake Mushrooms are another source, don't cook them, eat raw]

-Sulforaphane Glucosinolate You shouldn't need to supplement. [Cruciferous Vegetables]

-Thiamine Critical supplement for the thyroid. Many people get relief from chronic fatigue within a few days of taking thiamine. I suggest supplement + food sources for those having thyroid issues. [Yeast Extract, Seaweed, Flaxseed, Tahini]

-Turmeric, also called Curcumin. This is both a supplement (pill form, which I have never taken) and cooking spice (absolute staple in the NakedFood kitchen). I've dedicated a separate page for Turmeric, it's at the beginning of this Brain Food section, in case you skipped it.

-Vitamin D Sun is best, ever met a depressed surfer? If sun is impossible, then liquid, micellized is absorbed best.

-Vitamin E Liquid drops are easy to find, you shouldn't need to supplement if you have a strong diet. [Agar Seaweed, Dried Apricots, Avocado]

-Vitamin K 26% of people with Celiac Disease are usually deficient. Embrace parsley. Replace regular salad with Taboulleh (spelled a dozen ways, including Tabouli) for a while. CAREFUL: original version is made with cracked wheat ("bulgur"), so don't buy it at the grocery store. You can replace that with cooked quinoa or skip it altogether. Simple recipe (all finely chopped/diced): parsley, tomato, small onion, cucumber, mint, lemon, salt, olive oil. You can also get condensed parsley/kale/chard by using them in the dip recipes. [Parsley, Kale, Swiss Chard]

-Zinc (carnosine) Supplement if your system is overall low (as always, I don't like shooting blind and prefer knowing for sure with test results). Most people don't need to supplement once they're out of damage control, have strengthened, and are now in maintenance mode. [Shiitake Mushrooms, Agar Seaweed, Sesame/Tahini]

If you're not sure on brands, I have suggestions to the ones I personally use (I have no direct affiliation to any company, none of them sponsor me to suggest them) JaquiKarr.com/Resources

Ideally, we wouldn't supplement with anything, our rich food supply would give us everything we need. But our current state of affairs doesn't allow us that luxury. Do your best to get the most you can from foods and use supplements to do what their name says: supplement. Supplement a strong diet, don't use supplements as the only nutrition in your diet.

So critical, it's on a page of its own. Please read all the important tips, too many people are getting this wrong.

"While dietary intervention can induce significant change, it is possible that the level of impact may not always be sufficient to engineer the changes in microbial populations that are conducive to better health. The use of probiotics and other strategies may be required."[312]

A happy gut is the key to a lot of disorders, and probiotics (even in science labs) are proving to be the therapy of choice for every issue from IBS[313] to Autism[314].

If you're newly diagnosed, there's damage control to do, load up on supplements for 6-12 months. In maintenance mode, you can use any combination you like: Just pre/probiotic rich food, just supplements, or a mix of both. I do mix of both, it's just too important. Whether you get them through food or supplements, I'd suggest everyone make this a staple, your gut doesn't do well without probiotics, and that disrupts your brain and emotions.

FOODS: KOMBUCHA, SAUERKRAUT (or KIMCHI)

Kombucha Tea: You get a little starter kit and a big glass jug, very small initial investment. I know someone who has been making brews of kombucha, all feeding from a batch he started 3 years ago. My favorite part is having fun with flavors. I throw in 3 blueberries and the whole thing gets a pretty blue tint. Ginger is still my all-time favorite (maybe because it reminds me of champagne).

Sauerkraut (from German, sauer "sour" + Kraut "vegetable"): Again, a very small investment, all you need is that big pot you initially buy. Then it's all about vegetables, salt, squish, and wait. "Kimchi" is the same as sauerkraut, it's just the Korean name for it and traditionally uses more spices.

FOOD POWER TIP 1: I'm starting to see foods like chia enhanced with probiotics. Just be sure they're "live", and then be sure you keep them that way by not adding any heat to them. Store in fridge once you open the package.

FOOD POWER TIP 2: There are certain foods that are marketed to you as great sources of probiotics. They're not missing from this book by accident. Dairy (including Kefir) does more harm than good, so ignore all the sexy tummy yogurt commercials (5000 points to the Marketing Masters). Tempeh, seems legit, but this is a soy product. Besides most of the world's soy being GMO, soy is a thyroid disruptor. Miso (Japanese) is also soy based and the traditional way also includes barley (gluten) so it's out, big time.

BUYING SUPPLEMENTS

SUPPLEMENT POWER TIP 1: Be sure to take supplements with ultra-clean water (which means medical grade filter or reverse osmosis) because several common chemicals in tap water kill probiotics on contact and you completely defeat the purpose, might as well not take them at all. ...That should tell you something about drinking tap or plastic bottle water. If you can't afford a high-grade filter, get the hundred-dollar portable one I suggest at JaquiKarr.com/Resources

SUPPLEMENT POWER TIP 2: Each time you buy a probiotic, buy a new strain, finish the bottle, then buy another strain until you exhaust all good quality ones. Then start again from the beginning. Make sure Bifidobacteria and Lactobacillus are in at least one of the cycles you get (not necessarily both in the same bottle). The little we know is still barely the tip of the iceberg, but at least alternating bottles gives you the most of what's available to date. *Control what you can, don't stress what you can't.*

SUPPLEMENT POWER TIP 3: When to take them. There hasn't been a lot of research on this. Institut Rosell, which happens to be in my hometown of Montreal did an interesting experiment[315] re-creating the digestive tract with actual fluids. They found probiotics maintained their highest numbers when taken with fat, with meals, or up to 30 minutes before meals that included fat. Probiotics taken 30 minutes after meals had the lowest survival rates.

A FEW LAST THINGS

Mindset

Part of brain food is the right mindset and vantage point.

"Your body is attacking itself" is a description that needs to stop. It's how even the good guys are describing autoimmune disorders, and it's wrong.

The body NEVER attacks itself. If it did, you'd be dead in seconds. You actually think if your body wanted to shut down that you'd still be breathing? Are they kidding? The body is ALWAYS trying to protect you. ALWAYS. Always. ALWAYS. No-fail, all day, every day. We're just throwing too many wrenches in the wheel for it to keep up.

Every symptom you have is your body communicating to you and asking you for help. Your body doesn't have email, text, or cell phone access. The only way your body can communicate to you is via symptom.

If you think your body turned on you and it was or still is "attacking itself", then you're separating yourself from your body, and it's now the enemy. How conducive does that sound to healing? Sounds like a nuance, but it can make all the difference in the world.

Here's the mindset: Damn, our food supply is a mess and I accidentally got caught up in the spiderweb. Lucky for me, my body caught it and started sending signals, *thank you gorgeous genius body, I appreciate what you did for me, and now I'll do my part.*

No one is attacking anyone. We're working harmoniously to wellness. We're going **home** to **home**ostasis. *Together.*

If You Were My Best Friend...

...You *are* my best friend. You're a person I share our one planet with. When you're not well, we all, collectively, are slightly less well. I don't stay contained in my isolated bionic-healthy bubble and look at you from a space station. So, here are my last few words, off the record, from one friend to another.

Think of how many times you've heard the PhDs say: "We NOW know that..." and they proceed to tell us what we know today, which is the total opposite of what they thought they knew 2, 5, 10, 40 years ago. Gut bacteria used to be evil and needed sanitizing. A few short years later, gut bacteria is the secret to health and every health topic revolves around the gut microbiome.

That scenario will never stop. Humans thinking that they know what they're talking about is an infinite loop and it happens over and over, before each time that we blow ourselves up. At the rate we're going, we have 150-200 years before the next boom.

The undeniable truth is: We barely know anything, and we'll always barely know anything. Stop trusting humans, scientists, me, your grandmother... your cat is the wisest person in the room, until we figure out a way to completely kill its natural instincts too.

Trust Nature. Trust the process of photosynthesis:

1) Seed (you)
2) Sun (happy life choices, good relationships, fulfilling work)
3) Water (actual real pure water + real food / nourishment)

Source, Nature, doesn't matter what you call it: Never fails. Never. Humans fail. Humans fail every chance you give them. Why would you follow the failing team when you have one that's never been defeated? Even when we think we have it beat, all we do is blow ourselves up. Earth remains right where it is, regenerates, and starts all over... for the next set of humans to blow themselves up.

Trust the natural intelligence inside you. You know that chemically loaded, processed foods can't be right. You don't need studies to tell you that. Eat the foods you know are right and your brilliant body will do the rest.

Remember my tormented walk on the beach, as I was trying to figure out how I could possibly explain all this to others? You now have that same burden. You can make some points over drinks, but you can't really cover much ground by the 3rd round of martinis (cheers!) We have a serious epidemic on our hands, and the solution for our society is one thing: More informed people. Please do your part.

Please take 60 seconds and write a 5-star review from wherever you bought this book, then go on social media and share. Help others become as informed as you now are. It's not governments that are going to solve this, it's you and me. Thank you so very much.

Peace, Love, and Walnuts
-Jaqui Karr

P.S. There's still a ton of information for you in the 5 Bonus Chapters

P.P.S. If you need to be strictly gluten free, you'll want my A to Z list, details at JaquiKarr.com/Books

Health Professionals

Did you know that it's usually not a gastroenterologist who diagnoses Celiac[316]? And even when they do, it's usually after the person was unofficially diagnosed by someone like you. By a friend, a sharp health coach, a personal trainer who recognized symptoms, a nutritionist, a retailer in the supplements aisle, a naturopath out of ideas, a homeopath not getting results and suspecting toxins... it's almost always not a doctor that initially suspects gluten.

We're past the 11th hour and need more Health Professionals, of all types, to understand gluten at clinical levels and to know all its symptoms and how to easily spot a gluten sufferer.

I've created a course that gets you to my level of knowledge on this. No fluff, all substance, all science-based, like this book. You'll feel like you're in a live seminar with me.   Details at JaquiKarr.com/Gluten

Thank you for reading this book, you're already miles ahead of everyone else. And thanks in advance for leaving a review, they're incredibly important.
   -Jaqui

Bonus Chapters

1. **Beyond Food.** Movement, sleep, meditation are elements you can consider brain food.

2. **Most Common Gluten-Related Symptoms.** The well-known ones and the not-so-well known ones that are actually more common. Testing can be expensive and not-so-fun. You might want to use this as your 30 second quick check before deciding to go through formal testing. Ideally, after reading all this, you drop gluten.

3. **A full list of autoimmune disorders linked to gluten,** in case you're suspecting your issue is actually a symptom. This list includes the more obscure ones that aren't in the more common short lists I provide in chapter 2 of this section.

4. **Going Gluten Free.** Power tips and a few things not commonly discussed that might be helpful to you.

3. **Testing Methods and Checklists.** In case you'd like a formal diagnosis, plus additional information, including the advancements in Europe that we're not seeing in North America yet.

1. Beyond Food

This section contains 3 elements that I consider Brain Food:

1) Movement

2) Sleep

3) Meditation

I have complete and utter faith that you're eating fantastically. These 3 elements will elevate your health to the next level.

Movement (easy at-home solution)

Exercise increases BDNF (Brain Derived Neurotrophic Factor), renews brain cells and the connection between cells.

If you want to protect your brain, exercise. Over the long term, there's significantly less cognitive decline in those who enjoy a "high level of physical activity" (that's your best bet), but you're still protecting your brain with "low-to-moderate level exercise[317]" compared to no exercise at all.

> "Compared with no exercise, physical activity was associated with lower risks of cognitive impairment, Alzheimer disease, and dementia of any type."[318]

> "Women with higher levels of baseline physical activity were less likely to develop cognitive decline."[319]

Exercise is a form of brain food.

Ideally, I'd like to see your butt outdoors and enjoying Nature while brisk walking, jogging, paddling, kayaking, any-ing that's a verb... but I get it, not everyone's cup of tea. I've had plenty of clients tell me: "Look, I'm up at 6AM getting my kids ready, then work, soccer practice, dinner, and where am I supposed to leave my kids when I go to the gym?" Yes, I hear you...

THE EASIEST WAY TO WORK OUT

My best solution (for myself as well) are yoga videos. They're convenient, require no travel time, no gym membership expense, no equipment or special gear (all you need is a mat), and you have every level of workout and strength training you need.

Yoga is misunderstood as chanting OM and doing feeble stretches. Think again. After 20 years of yoga, I still can't do many poses, they're just too hard for me. You can develop a dancer's or surfer's body doing 30 minutes of yoga, 5 days a week (preferably every day). My personal regimen is every day, until my body says to break. Every few weeks I'll get a day that feels like I was weight-training too hard (from yoga!) and I take the day off to let my muscle recover. I never schedule days off, I wait until I feel it.

197

Some sequences are fast enough to get a cardio workout. Others are slow, intense poses that are challenging enough to get toning that rivals weight training (minus the wear & tear on joints and cartilage). Get the right program and style, and you'll be shocked at what a beach body you can have.

The DVD's I live and die by are at JaquiKarr.com/Resources

These DVD's are still the only exercise that I have done consistently for 20 years. Everything else, even running, I do in phases, with seasons, influenced by travel, etc. But I never skip yoga. I travel with my DVD's and play them on laptop if needed. Yoga keeps me toned, physically and mentally.

POWER TIPS

1) If you're a total beginner, it might be hard to keep up with even basic sequences. Go into it accepting that you won't get through a single workout fluidly for several weeks. When I started, I was no stranger to working out and it still took me a month to get through a 25-minute sequence (and this still happens when I start new programs... not a month anymore, but it can take several days to get straight through a new sequence). Focus on form, the rest will come.

2) Stick to one instructor for a while. Variety is fun, but not while you're learning. Every instructor has their style, you don't need to get spun in circles. Many rename poses from the original Sanskrit name, which is helpful, "tree pose" is easier to remember than "Vrksasana", but not every instructor might say tree pose. They might call it something else, and by the time you look at them and figure that out, they're on to the next move and you're frustrated. Stick to one instructor until you have the basics down and you're getting a good workout and enjoying it, then experiment if you like.

3) Stop the video when needed. Nothing says you need to do an entire sequence while you're learning poses. Stop the video, practice the pose your instructor is on several times, until you feel you have the posture right. These poses are all new to your muscles and they'll need to be trained (See? You're getting weight training effect already). Instead of doing 30 poses terribly and feeling frustrated, do 5 poses well by stopping the video and doing them over and over. Then add one by one, as your energy and time allow. No pressure. Breathe :) It's yoga, not the trading floor on Wall Street.

Yoga is brain *and* soul food. *Namaste.*

Sleep

Sleep is the maintenance that a race car needs. Notice how many crew members take care of race cars? Things need to repair, entire tires need to be changed, oil added, all kinds of things happen. That's your body. All kinds of things need to change, renew, regenerate. It all happens while you're sleeping. You can't change a car tire while you're still driving the car.

The science on sleep is overwhelming, but we don't need science to tell us what we already know is great for us. All I'll say is: You, my dear Ferrari, need to make sure you respect what a powerful machine you are and take good care.

7-8 hours solid sleep is what to aim for. More if your body tells you it needs more. You might need to re-arrange both work and personal habits for this to happen, it's worth it.

RITUAL CAN HELP

You've probably read articles ranging from warm bath before bed to counting sheep, I won't repeat what you've already seen a hundred times. Figuring out a ritual can have a Pavlovian effect on signaling your system that it's time for sleep.

A few minutes of meditation or breath work can do wonders for your sleeping ritual. Calming sounds and scents are both helpful. I love ocean waves *(there's a shocker)*, but sometimes after harrowing days, travel, 22 non-stop hours of work, I put on the Schumann Resonance (the earth's core sound, good thing to reconnect to). As far as audios go, you have a lot of options from the beautiful chants of monks (who have many audios out) to guided meditations, to soothing classical, and on it goes.

WHAT TO AVOID:

1) Hyper-stimulating or violent movies and music.

2) The news. Hasn't changed, *ever.* I turned off news 15 years ago, couldn't tell you who the anchors on any news program are. When a plane falls from the sky, don't worry, someone will tell you... and that will be an actual conversation with a humanoid.

3) Social Media, can be worse than news (usually just a condensed feed of news). At least CNN doesn't send you hate mail or bully kids. Contain what you see to actual friends, not insanity.
BTW, a lot of you (awesome cool folks, I love you sincerely) are killing me asking me to post and be visible online again. Creates a genuine dilemma because I'd be 100% offline if there weren't so many of you who are great, and if your success stories from my online info didn't keep coming in. Please tell me this book, written as raw as I've ever written, provided connection?

4) Cell phone. I shut mine off at 9 p.m. (or earlier) unless I have a pre-scheduled call, usually that's from a different time zone. It's unbelievable, but somehow, the world manages to go on without me answering texts immediately. Sun, moon, and stars continue to do their thing too ;)

5) WIFI Signals. Do turn off all WIFI in the house before going to bed. Your neighbors' signals are bad enough, cut down on the ones closest to your bed (and brain). Besides the radio waves themselves, for your sanity (and anxiety levels), limit how much time you spend online altogether. Structure set times to check emails instead of getting constant notifications. Turn off all notifications that are unnecessary for your work and check messages once or twice a day, or less. Learn to disconnect and get off the grid every night, even if it can't be in wild terrain and under billions of twinkling stars.

Are there exceptions? Sure. If you're an emergency doctor on call, you can't turn off your phone and it needs to be by your bed. Are you someone that needs to be reached 24/7? I have a friend with a chain of restaurants, while not an E.R. doctor, he certainly has his fair share of emergencies. If you truly need to stay connected, you know the policy: Do the best with what you can control, don't stress what you can't.

NAPPING

Most people immediately say "impossible". Alright, hold on, let's look at that. Is it truly impossible?

Do you work in an office? Most people get an afternoon coffee break. Can you go lie in your car, with an alarm set, and use your coffee break to nap? Lunch. Can you take a late lunch? Instead of noon, you take 1 or 2 p.m., use half an hour to eat your lunch and the rest of the time to lie in your car or under a tree, if weather permits and you have access. Cafeteria gossip will damage your brain, napping will strengthen it.

On the road salesperson? You definitely can nap. I've done it in concrete parking lots with ocean waves running on my headphones (get stereo, noise-cancelling, full ear muffs).

Impossible isn't always impossible. It just seems that way as a first gut reaction, especially if your schedule is hectic. The more hectic your schedule, the more a nap can probably help you. Do a Costanza under your desk if you have to, find a way to nap.

The Japanese have sleep pods at most of their corporate offices. They've known for decades that the brain rejuvenates and functions better when it gets some down time outside of regular sleep time.

NIGHT OWLS / NIGHT SHIFT WORKERS / CIRCADIAN RHYTHM

Every living thing on earth (including us) works with light and dark, we're wired with sun and moon and *I won't get too esoteric.* Think of all the plants and flowers that literally open up and put their face up to the sun, then close completely through the night.

If you're in night work / shift work, make sure you're taking measures like installing total blackout curtains when you sleep (or eye mask, that's a $2 solution), get special lamps (many are made for SAD: Seasonal Affective Disorder) and put it by your desk at night to mimic daylight.

I put myself through school while working nights, and I did the zombie walk for many years, so believe me, I'm not criticizing. If you make your living working off-hours, it is what it is. Compensate the best you can.

> "All studies reported significant findings or trends towards significance in a broad range of measures, including a reduction of cognitive decline, reduction in perceived stress, increase in quality of life, as well as increases in functional connectivity, percent volume brain change and cerebral blood flow in areas of the cortex."[320]

We're in relatively early stages of measuring brains that meditate, but the results are consistent: "These preliminary results indicate that in adults with MCI [mild cognitive impairment], MBSR [Mindfulness Based Stress Reduction] may have a positive impact on the regions of the brain most related to MCI and AD [Alzheimer's Disease]."[321]

Meditation has "positive effects on telomere regulation."[322]

They're even seeing that meditation can be used to improve gut health: "Meditation helps regulate the stress response, thereby suppressing chronic inflammation states and maintaining a healthy gut-barrier function."[323]

It can be a challenging habit at first, not just in terms of making the time for it, but actually sitting still and silent.

POWER TIPS

1) Don't assume you're supposed to achieve a totally blank mind, you don't need the pressure of getting to Buddha status within a week. Your mind will wander, that's fine, gently bring it back. Don't beat yourself up about it, don't get annoyed and quit. You might even learn more about yourself by noticing patterns. If your mind keeps drifting to the same issue, maybe you need to make a change in your life regarding that issue.

2) Mantras can be helpful. You repeat a sound or a phrase, and by focusing on that sound, it forces your focus away from everything else. It also creates a rhythmic calmness that comes with music, and there's no reason we can't consider mantras/chanting to be a form of music (Have you heard the chants of monks? You can buy them as audio programs).

3) Guided meditations are excellent for beginners. Some argue that it defeats the point of total blankness. Maybe. But focusing on one sound is a lot more progress than 20,000 thoughts, grocery list, to-do list, weekend plans, work issues, ... I can meditate well on my own after 25 years, yet I still use guided meditations sometimes because they're so soothing and sometimes it's a message I needed to hear.

4) Movement meditation might be a great option for some. I took Tai Chi lessons in Korea years ago and can tell you that was pure meditation. So are certain yoga practices. I have a yoga DVD entirely focused on meditation, both with and without movement. Link at JaquiKarr.com/Resources and I'll also add a link to the best book I've read for beginners on meditation.

I'm paraphrasing and don't know who to credit this to, but it sums it up nicely:
Person: "I don't have an hour to meditate every day."
Monk: "I see. That means you must meditate for 2 hours."
:)

Start with 5 minutes, take it from there. Commit to adding minutes until you're at 30 minutes at least. No pressure, as you're ready. Might take you months to get to 15 minutes, that's fine. Everything is perfectly fine, all is well. One extra minute is progress.

2. Most Common Gluten-Related Symptoms

THE WELL-KNOWN SYMPTOMS

"Classic Celiac", are the symptoms that will point to your gut:

❖ Bloating
❖ Cramps
❖ Diarrhea
❖ Discomfort after eating
❖ Gas
❖ Oily stool

These are all common in IBS, don't let your doctor convince you that you have IBS, that's usually a symptom, not a disease, which some studies are starting to recognize.

NOT-SO-FAMOUS SYMPTOMS, BUT MORE COMMON THAN CLASSIC CD

Symptoms the media hasn't focused on yet and haven't made famous:

- ❖ Abnormal weight (gain when it triggers thyroid or loss when it creates malabsorption)
- ❖ ADD / ADHD / focus issues / Autism (anywhere on the spectrum for all of them)
- ❖ Anorexia
- ❖ Back Pain
- ❖ Chronic Fatigue
- ❖ Dental decay
- ❖ Depression
- ❖ Erectile Dysfunction
- ❖ Hair Loss
- ❖ Headaches
- ❖ Infertility
- ❖ Insomnia
- ❖ Joint Pain
- ❖ Liver Disease
- ❖ Migraines
- ❖ Miscarriage
- ❖ Mood Swings
- ❖ Muscle Atrophy
- ❖ Osteoporosis and all bone deterioration
- ❖ Skin disorders (ALL skin disorders: eczema, psoriasis, dermatitis herpetiformis)
- ❖ Thyroid malfunction
- ❖ Vitamin Deficiencies (and all the issues that opens you up to)

Gluten related damage can be neurological, endocrine, combinations of issues, and of course digestive complications and the spin-off problems that are a result of not absorbing food and water properly.

These seemingly non-food related issues are often symptoms that become mystery issues and keep people sick for years and years, suffering needlessly, and often suffering to their death. It's heart breaking. You don't need to be that person.

3. List of Autoimmune and Autoimmune-Related Diseases

Autoimmune and Autoimmune-Related Diseases, as listed by The American Autoimmune Related Diseases Association[324]

Acute Disseminated Encephalomyelitis (ADEM)
Acute necrotizing hemorrhagic leukoencephalitis
Addison's disease
Agammaglobulinemia
Alopecia areata
Amyloidosis
Ankylosing spondylitis
Anti-GBM/Anti-TBM nephritis
Antiphospholipid syndrome (APS)
Autoimmune angioedema
Autoimmune aplastic anemia
Autoimmune dysautonomia
Autoimmune hepatitis
Autoimmune hyperlipidemia
Autoimmune immunodeficiency
Autoimmune inner ear disease (AIED)
Autoimmune myocarditis
Autoimmune oophoritis
Autoimmune pancreatitis
Autoimmune retinopathy
Autoimmune thrombocytopenic purpura (ATP)
Autoimmune thyroid disease
Autoimmune urticaria
Axonal & neuronal neuropathies
Balo disease
Behcet's disease
Bullous pemphigoid
Cardiomyopathy
Castleman disease
Celiac disease
Chagas disease
Chronic fatigue syndrome**
Chronic inflammatory demyelinating polyneuropathy (CIDP)
Chronic recurrent multifocal ostomyelitis (CRMO)
Churg-Strauss syndrome
Cicatricial pemphigoid/benign mucosal pemphigoid
Crohn's disease
Cogans syndrome
Cold agglutinin disease
Congenital heart block
Coxsackie myocarditis

CREST disease
Essential mixed cryoglobulinemia
Demyelinating neuropathies
Dermatitis herpetiformis
Dermatomyositis
Devic's disease (neuromyelitis optica)
Discoid lupus
Dressler's syndrome
Endometriosis
Eosinophilic esophagitis
Eosinophilic fasciitis
Erythema nodosum
Experimental allergic encephalomyelitis
Evans syndrome
Fibromyalgia**
Fibrosing alveolitis
Giant cell arteritis (temporal arteritis)
Giant cell myocarditis
Glomerulonephritis
Goodpasture's syndrome
Granulomatosis with Polyangiitis (GPA) (formerly called Wegener's Granulomatosis)
Graves' disease
Guillain-Barre syndrome
Hashimoto's encephalitis
Hashimoto's thyroiditis
Hemolytic anemia
Henoch-Schonlein purpura
Herpes gestationis
Hypogammaglobulinemia
Idiopathic thrombocytopenic purpura (ITP)
IgA nephropathy
IgG4-related sclerosing disease
Immunoregulatory lipoproteins
Inclusion body myositis
Interstitial cystitis
Juvenile arthritis
Juvenile diabetes (Type 1 diabetes)
Juvenile myositis
Kawasaki syndrome
Lambert-Eaton syndrome
Leukocytoclastic vasculitis
Lichen planus
Lichen sclerosus
Ligneous conjunctivitis
Linear IgA disease (LAD)

Lupus (SLE)
Lyme disease, chronic
Meniere's disease
Microscopic polyangiitis
Mixed connective tissue disease (MCTD)
Mooren's ulcer
Mucha-Habermann disease
Multiple sclerosis
Myasthenia gravis
Myositis
Narcolepsy
Neuromyelitis optica (Devic's)
Neutropenia
Ocular cicatricial pemphigoid
Optic neuritis
Palindromic rheumatism
PANDAS (Pediatric Autoimmune Neuropsychiatric Disorders Associated with Streptococcus)
Paraneoplastic cerebellar degeneration
Paroxysmal nocturnal hemoglobinuria (PNH)
Parry Romberg syndrome
Parsonnage-Turner syndrome
Pars planitis (peripheral uveitis)
Pemphigus
Peripheral neuropathy
Perivenous encephalomyelitis
Pernicious anemia
POEMS syndrome
Polyarteritis nodosa
Type I, II, & III autoimmune polyglandular syndromes
Polymyalgia rheumatica
Polymyositis
Postmyocardial infarction syndrome
Postpericardiotomy syndrome
Progesterone dermatitis
Primary biliary cirrhosis
Primary sclerosing cholangitis
Psoriasis
Psoriatic arthritis
Idiopathic pulmonary fibrosis
Pyoderma gangrenosum
Pure red cell aplasia
Raynauds phenomenon
Reactive Arthritis
Reflex sympathetic dystrophy
Reiter's syndrome

Relapsing polychondritis
Restless legs syndrome
Retroperitoneal fibrosis
Rheumatic fever
Rheumatoid arthritis
Sarcoidosis
Schmidt syndrome
Scleritis
Scleroderma
Sjogren's syndrome
Sperm & testicular autoimmunity
Stiff person syndrome
Subacute bacterial endocarditis (SBE)
Susac's syndrome
Sympathetic ophthalmia
Takayasu's arteritis
Temporal arteritis/Giant cell arteritis
Thrombocytopenic purpura (TTP)
Tolosa-Hunt syndrome
Transverse myelitis
Type 1 diabetes
Ulcerative colitis
Undifferentiated connective tissue disease (UCTD)
Uveitis
Vasculitis
Vesiculobullous dermatosis
Vitiligo
Wegener's granulomatosis (now termed Granulomatosis with Polyangiitis (GPA)

NOTE: Fibromyalgia and Chronic Fatigue are listed, not because they are autoimmune, but because many persons who suffer from them have associated autoimmune disease(s)

TESTING FOR HASHIMOTO'S

TSH misses Hashimoto's in early stages by up to 10-15 years, depending on speed of degeneration.

SOLUTION is to look for thyroid antibodies, which will show up in early stages, before unnecessary damage goes too far:

1) Thyroid peroxidase antibody (TPO)
   (for Hashimoto's and Graves)

2) Thyroglobulin antibody (TGAb)

MEASURING GENERAL THYROID FUNCTION

1) Free T3
2) Free T4

FOODS TO AVOID WITH THYROID ISSUES: Soy, Gluten, Dairy

Have you noticed it's always the same 5 offenders? Hundreds of diseases and it always comes back to gluten, dairy, sugar, soy, artificial fats / oils / sweeteners.

4. Going Gluten Free

Priority #1: Be certain gluten isn't sneaking its way onto your plate if you're reacting at clinical levels. That includes the legal 20PPM (not in all countries, some are higher, others are lower). Bonus report "20 PPMs and Other Gluten Roulette Numbers" is in this section.

If you're going gluten free simply as a choice (this means you've tested negative for all gluten antibodies, not just official CD testing), then you don't need to be as concerned about the small traces of cross contamination in restaurants as someone who is reacting acutely needs to be (which is a massive lifestyle difference, and a non-returning rocket you don't want to launch).

Beyond that, here are some pointers that will help you as you cross over to the GF side of life...

Toe Dip vs Deep Dive

For someone who has a lot to say on the topic, in person, you'd be shocked at how quiet of a person I am. I was at a V.I.P. party at a large conference recently. Thousands of attendees, maybe a little over a 150 people or so at this party. Many of them were functional medicine doctors, a practice I appreciate.

They were talking about ways to slowly help their patients with diet change. Some of them had developed year-long plans. Others would make one change, then explore a second at the 6-month check-up. I silently listened for almost an hour at all the different strategies they were using to try to get patients to eat better, and many of them had in-house nutritionists with strategies of their own.

One of the doctors was someone I had previously done consulting for, he knew my track record. He noticed I wasn't contributing to their discussion and finally he asked, "How do you do it? Your results are unparalleled. Have you found an ideal time frame to transition people to healthier habits?"

My answer stopped the proverbial music... you know that moment in movies when the whole party stops and gets quiet? My answer was: "I've never figured out how to transition someone out of a burning house over a period of a year. I see fire, I don't even take the time to yell fire, I get them out immediately and work on their burn marks."

Dive. I'll catch you.

COMMITMENT CREATES AND MAINTAINS HEALING

One of the things that put me on stage was my phenomenally quick recovery after being in as serious a condition as I was. It wasn't that I was a genius, it's that I knew to tap into Nature's genius. Once I knew gluten was the issue, the rest was easy.

I was running 10 miles a day again only 90 days after my last E.R. visit, which needed an I.V. to keep me conscious. Remarkable? Not really. But I didn't go to the grocery store and buy every gluten-free labeled box, adding different toxins to my blood.

I went on an all green juice diet for the first 6 weeks, and I went to Home Depot for aloe vera plants. I bought up every aloe plant from the gardening section and made them order cases more.

Every morning, I cut a leaf and squeezed aloe gel into my drink. Every evening, I squeezed aloe gel into my martini shaker, added pure cranberry or pomegranate juice, ice, *shaken not stirred,* and had cocktail hour. That's how I healed my gut faster. If you followed me in earlier days, that's what the martini in my original logo was about. It was my nightly, very civilized, cocktail hour. The martini glass was good for morale too, it didn't feel clinical. To succeed at this, you have to be fully immersed and make it a part of your lifestyle and do whatever little things you need to do to feel good about it. *Salud.*

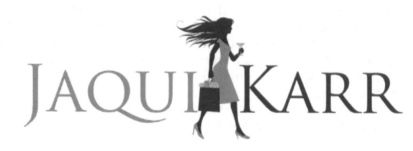

"20 Ppms and Other Gluten Roulette Numbers"

I took a hard hit for this when I first published it. Since then, I've received messages from a lot of people telling me it was the one missing piece of the puzzle that got them to 100% wellness.

GRAS (Generally Regarded As Safe) protects industry, it doesn't help the public. A little cyanide won't kill most people... but does that make it a good idea to keep consuming small amounts?

I'll start with the Bottom Line: There is no study in the world that conclusively finds any amount of gluten safe for Celiac Disease. They find it "generally" safe and "most can tolerate" (I already went into detail on that in a previous chapter). But no study can (ethically) conclude any amount of gluten is safe for all Celiacs.

I understand business. I understand how devastating it would be for almost every gluten free food manufacturer in the world if the law said 0 gluten to be certified gluten free…. Though this hasn't stopped Australia, they're champions for how they've regulated requirements for Certified GF. If Australia can do it, so can the rest of the world.
It's time for business to understand life. Life is short. Life is precious. It's not meant to be lived in disease. If a company can't do 0 gluten, get out of the gluten free game and cater to standard diets. Simple.

Our History is a History of Cover Ups:

-Cigarettes were "safe" for 60 years while there were studies showing disease from day 1

-GMO's and chemicals on foods show horrific 3-headed frogs and fish that change sex in studies, and still legally Generally Regarded As Safe

-Vaccine injury payouts surpassed 3 Billion dollars years ago, yet vaccines are all deemed GRAS and doctors (the few who know the truth) are petrified to speak up. No one wants to be "Wakefielded" (A verb that shouldn't exist, the crushing of Dr. Wakefield, only for suggesting the link between vaccines and autism should be studied. He didn't even make a definitive statement. He didn't have Oprah's money and notoriety to come out of it on top.)

So now here we go again. The studies are showing us that there is no safe amount of gluten for people reacting to gluten (I'm sure no more of those will be funded). Should we start a pool on how many decades it will take for government to admit it? I have $10 on 55 years. The pro-wheat campaign is already heavily under way, with trillions of dollars behind them.

Clearly, I have a lot more to say on this issue, but I won't. The facts speak for themselves. It's up to health care professionals to share facts and let the consumer make their choices. Informed choices.

Someone once told me "I don't care what happens to me, I'm not giving up bread." I respect that. It falls under "consenting adults" in my book, and I live my life under the code of "Live and Let Live". I'm only here to inform, final decisions fall on each individual. Make an informed decision, look at these studies...

[My personal comments are preceded with "JK", to differentiate my words from the studies]

STUDY 1[325]: "...the daily amount of gluten that can be safely consumed is not yet defined"

"RECENT FINDINGS: Gluten-free diet is generally admitted as effective therapy in symptomatic patients, but a life-long dietary treatment in some challenging cases such as 'silent' and 'latent' patients is under discussion.

Tolerance to gluten may be acquired later in life, but, as latency may be transient, a strict follow-up is necessary in these patients. The composition of gluten-free diet needs a better definition; latest evidence demonstrates that oats are tolerated by most patients with coeliac disease.

Finally, the amount of gluten permitted in gluten-free products is still a matter of debate; significant progress has been made in the sensitivity of techniques for gluten detection, but the daily amount of gluten that can be safely consumed is not yet defined."

STUDY 2[326]: "...there is no evidence to suggest a single definitive threshold"

214

"RESULTS: Thirteen studies (three randomized controlled, one cohort, two crossover, and seven cross-sectional) met the inclusion criteria. The daily amount of tolerable gluten varied widely between studies. Whilst some patients tolerated an average of 34-36 mg of gluten per day, other patients who consumed about 10 mg of gluten per day developed mucosal abnormalities. The effect of the consumption of 'glutenfree' products with different degrees of gluten contamination was also inconsistent.

CONCLUSIONS: The amount of tolerable gluten varies among people with coeliac disease. Although there is no evidence to suggest a single definitive threshold, a daily gluten intake of <10 mg is unlikely to cause significant histological abnormalities."

JK: "Unlikely to cause..."??? They're handling gluten the way they handle vaccines: if it kills or paralyzes only a minority of people, then it's not a significant enough risk for them to stop it. But what about the lower levels of damage? Depression, chronic fatigue, infertility... the issues that won't kill you instantly or put you in the hospital, but they will steal life itself from you.

STUDY 3[327]: "the sensitivity to trace intakes of gluten showed large interpatient variability"
"In conclusion, this study confirmed that an abnormal small-bowel morphology persisted in a significant proportion of CD patients being treated with a GFD, most likely because of the persistent ingestion of trace amounts of gluten. The protracted intake of 50 mg gluten/d produced significant damage in the architecture of the small intestine in patients being treated for CD.
However, the sensitivity to trace intakes of gluten showed large interpatient variability, a feature that should be accounted for in the implementation of a safe gluten threshold. These findings should be confirmed by further studies in larger numbers of CD patients. Finally, the relation between the intestinal damage induced by trace intakes of gluten and the long-term complications of CD remains to be elucidated."

JK: Several people had to be dropped every step of the way during the study due to intolerable pain or apparent damage being caused. Here are direct quotes from the study:

-"4 of 49 subjects had to be excluded from the protocol because severe enteropathy"

215

-"Furthermore, one patient challenged with 10 mg gluten/d experienced clinical symptoms after a few weeks, whereas none of the 13 subjects receiving 50 mg gluten/d had clinical evidence of relapse."

-"One patient (challenged with 10 mg gluten) developed a clinical relapse."

-"7 of the 49 patients had to be excluded because of abnormal small-intestinal histology, development of thyroid carcinoma, or gastric polyposis confirmed by gastroduodenoscopy or because the subject refused randomization."

-"One patient challenged with 10 mg gluten/d showed typical signs of relapse (vomiting, diarrhea, and abdominal distension) after 6-8 wk of microchallenge but refused to repeat the t1 evaluation."

JK: Dropped from the study means they never finished it... which means they got excluded from the conclusion. Yes, that's legal. "Where Science Meets Common Sense" ... if patients had to be dropped due to excruciating pain from a few drops of gluten, some hospitalized, shouldn't they be the first people mentioned in the conclusion?

They're also not counting the "gluten load". A patient might be able to ingest 10mg in one slice of supposed gluten free bread, but if they eat 2 slices of toast at breakfast + 2 slices in their sandwich at lunch + 2 buns with burger at dinner = 60mg or more. The studies conveniently talk about the minimum threshold, but who eats one tiny piece in an entire day when they're told that loaf is "certified gluten free"?

Zero gluten: that's what is safe.

If you realize you need to be strictly gluten free, use my A to Z list (JaquiKarr.com/Books) to check ingredients. I researched every item from scratch and this isn't an upsell. I think we both know I won't be retiring on a $5 item. I spent a year creating this list to keep you and I safe. Truly safe, not just minimum legal standards, and not the same list everyone has been copying from one web site to another. I also point out some ingredients that are gluten free, but exceptionally toxic.

Naturally Safe GF Flours

Note: corn, oats, and other foods normally listed as safe have been omitted because we have studies showing people reacting. This is your no-fail gluten free flour list

All Beans (use strong herbs / spices, you'll never taste bean)
All Nuts
All Seeds
Banana Flour (popping up everywhere)
Buckwheat
Cassava
Chick Pea (excellent for flatbreads and pizza crusts)
Coconut (lower in calories than nut flours for desserts)
Hemp
Lentil (cooks extremely fast, good for thin crusts or crackers)
Quinoa*
Wine flour

*Quinoa has a cross-contamination issue and a secondary issue no one is talking about... Popularity and demand for quinoa is growing, so you have some North American wheat farmers converting their crops to quinoa. That's soil that's been growing wheat for decades, which is why some samples have tested positive for gluten, it's not just a cross-contamination problem.

SOLUTION: Research brands that are either coming from South America, where it's been quinoa on that soil since the beginning, or safe North American soil that was growing potatoes or vegetables before planting quinoa. Research once, stick to that brand(s).

POWER TIP: You'll see more gluten free flours appearing in the coming years. GF demand keeps growing, which means so will supply. I expect to see some interesting foods being used to make flour (wine was novel, so was banana). It's all good. Just don't opt for flours that used gluten containing products to begin with and claim they're gluten free because of some type of processing. Whatever processing it took to (maybe) get gluten out, probably killed all nutrients with it. And legal parameters will allow for GRAS amounts of gluten to remain in those products. You have good options, don't roll the dice or go for cheap hyper-processed fillers.

HAVE PATIENCE

A lot of this is experimenting. I'm too raw to offer the best cooking advice, but of the times I've played:

Sweets: I've found almond flour great for cakes and cookies, and it provides a rich sweetness. Coconut flour is great for thick texture and absorbing other flavors.

Savory: I like chick pea or quinoa flour, depending on how thick of a texture I want. When I'm re-creating old fashioned pizza or a flatbread that I'm going to put on a hot stone, I use chick pea. For thin and crispy, I use quinoa or lentil flour.

Need recipes? I'll give you 10,000+ free ones. Go to Pinterest.ca/JaquiKarr and I challenge you to get through everything from just 3 of my boards in less than 25 years (Gluten-Free, Raw Food, Raw Desserts). The GF board is cooked recipes. Please note: I do my best to vet recipes but I'm sure some of them need some modifications (for sweeteners or artificial ingredients), and hopefully none have slipped through the cracks containing gluten. Always check ingredients against my A to Z list.

You'll botch up a few recipes until you get the hang of it, so what? Those make for the funniest stories. Though the fire department wasn't laughing when the neighbors once called because I set all the fire detectors off...

"Um, sorry to have bothered you. It wasn't me that dialed 911, there's no fire, just some smoke. I'm a raw girl you see, so I'm not used to baking, but I felt like having pizza and didn't realize lentil flour cooks a hundred times faster than wheat flour..."

It's all good. No one was hurt. Maybe one less cat had to find its own way out of a tree.

Gluten Withdrawals, Dairy & Autism

Withdrawals can happen when you get off gluten and/or all grains. Luckily, it's not as bad as getting off a morphine addiction, but wheat binds to receptors in your brain just like morphine and heroin[328], so you can possibly have symptoms.

You *might* feel a wide range of symptoms from headache to nausea, tough it out, it'll pass. And since you know it's (possibly) coming, you won't think something really bad is happening. Not everyone will go through withdrawals, this is just a precautionary section. Health Coaches: Please warn your clients so they don't panic should they get symptoms.

POWER TIPS

1) Don't over-exert. This is one of the few times when strenuous exercise is counter-productive. Detox takes a lot from your body, be in restful mode so all your energy is diverted to where it's needed. Get into a steam or sauna if you want to sweat things out and help detox along. Lighter walks are better than cardio work.

2) Leg pain or light-headed: Add some salt to food.

3) Hydrate. *Of course.* 2-3 liters of clean plastic-free water.

4) Coconut Water. Electrolytes are always a good thing, but especially good when your body needs all the help it can get. Chlorophyll in water can also help tremendously.

5) Don't wean off slowly, it doesn't work. As long as your brain is getting doses of grain-chemical hits, you're an addict. Get off the grain opiates and focus on new fantastic foods to keep your mind and mouth busy.

Some people suggest a long list of supplements and medical-grade herbs during withdrawals. I don't, because:

1) Your body still needs to process those, and it's busy enough. This isn't like standard detox.

2) Withdrawals usually don't last more than a few days, if at all. Longest one I've known in my experience was 6 days, they had flu-like symptoms and sweating and shaking, bad enough to be off work for a few days. Get under a cozy blanket, read a book, nap, have movie-marathons, let it pass on its own. If you sweat, shower a lot and get it off your skin. Drink lots and lots of water.

Notice how withdrawals don't happen when you stop eating any fruit or vegetable, or even meat. They only happen with grains, processed sugar, and dairy. Dairy has addictive morphine in it, "caso-morphin", built in by Nature. It's meant to keep the little calf safe and close to their mother so they don't drift off into danger and to potential predators. It's not meant to keep humans hostage to a harmful food.

CASOMORPHIN AND AUTISM

The more casomorphin, the more severe the autism symptoms, as found by mental health researchers in Russia. They also find casomorphin makes a normal child more susceptible to developing autism (shouldn't that be on the news?):

"Elevated concentrations of circulating casomorphins (CM), the exogenous opioid peptides from milk casein... The severity of autistic symptoms correlated with concentrations of CM-7 in the urine. Because CMs interact with opioid and serotonin receptors, the known modulators of synaptogenesis, we suggest that chronic exposure to elevated levels of bovine CMs may impair early child development, setting the stage for autistic disorders."[329]

GET HELP IF YOU NEED IT, WITHDRAWALS OR NOT

Emotional support is monumental (isn't that true for everything in life?) But with a diet change that feels radical to a lot of people, outside support, whether it's personal or professional can be the difference between sticking to the Gluten Free Lifestyle or slipping and suffering the consequences. "Psychological support seems to be able to reduce depression and to increase gluten-free diet compliance."[330]

Don't be shy to put up your hand and ask for help, and don't feel like you're being weak. Right in the medical books and studying thousands of case studies, we see that CD/NCGS runs far deeper than just the food factor. You weren't crazy with the things you were feeling pre-diagnosis, you're not crazy with what you're feeling now.

If we were meant to be alone, we'd all have our own island. Ask for help. You'd gladly lend a hand to someone you care about. Call a friend and say "I need girl time! This whole gluten thing is making me crazy," or "Dude, let's do something, I gotta get my mind off this food stuff" (just don't go for regular beers after that).

If you can afford it and feel comfortable, you may want to consider professional help too. I used to eat gluten regularly, but I was mostly focused on greens and very high raw when I got diagnosed, so going GF wasn't a big stretch for me. And I obviously knew too much about food to panic, I had replacements in my mind long before I needed them.

For others, it can be traumatic and feel devastating. If that's you, get whatever support you can, just be weary of online groups that do nothing but complain. I understand their frustration, but it's not the solution. Seek out support that can offer you some empathy, maybe even sympathy (we do need it sometimes to not feel alone and to feel understood), but overall, it's usually just an ear we need until adjusting to a new lifestyle. You don't want to get caught up in a perpetual complain group that never ends. You want to move on with your life, in a new and improved way.

Colonics

Welcome to the sexy portion of this book :)

Colonics (also called hydrotherapy) are the fast-forward button to wellness. It's part of the daily regimen in many holistic healing centers around the world. But there's a right and wrong way.

The knee-jerk conclusion is you're washing out bad bacteria, but good bacteria as well, so colonics are bad. Terrible conclusion. Funny how none of those people worry about the acid-wash you're getting before doing a colonoscopy and getting a camera crawling through you. We're just talking clean water here and it's troublesome?

Yes, you're washing everything out, but that's a good thing. Right there on the table, after treatment, you get a power dose of a probiotic enema (and now it doesn't have a mess of bad guys to fight, it can directly do its job on a clean canvas and heal you faster). I did a week of colonics immediately after diagnoses.

If your body's a disaster, chances are you aren't going to absorb probiotics too well orally anyways. This is ultimately the best way to get things on track instantly. TIP: I see some experts suggesting probiotic enemas at home, I'm not a fan of this. Do it if you're really comfortable with it, but know that you can hurt yourself (especially men) if you insert too deep. These are the kinds of things I personally leave to qualified professionals.

The trick to colonics is to find a good clinic. Do not go to beauty spas unless they have a true health expert / naturopath / nurse / etc. doing the treatment. For heaven's sake, do not do it yourself (called "open" treatment). Egyptian hieroglyphics and drawings clearly show them doing colonics, and I'm betting it wasn't self-applied then either.

CHECKLIST OF QUESTIONS

1) Who is doing the treatment, are they certified therapists, how many years have they been doing colonics? (At least a year.)

2) Is your system open or closed? (Avoid open.)

3) Does the technician/therapist/whatever-their-title stay with me from beginning to end? (I've come across places where a nurse is moving room to room with multiple people in the middle of treatment, it's insane. They make 3x more money, you get 3x less attention, and if she's delayed by a few seconds, you might find yourself in severe pain with water overload, and potentially dangerous issues.)

4) How long does the session last? (Under 40 minutes means they're not being thorough.)

5) Do you provide probiotic enemas after treatment? (If no, find another clinic.)

6) How is the water filtered? (A fluffy spa will use tap water. A proper establishment will have a high-end water filter, ensuring maximum purity.)

POWER TIPS

1) Don't do just one, that's dangerous. If you plan to do only one, I strongly suggest you do none. You're excavating years' worth of toxins, and then they have nowhere to go, so they flood your bloodstream. People have ended up in toxic shock and in emergency rooms from this. Uncommon, but it happens.

If it's your first time, do at least 5 or 6, maximum 48 hours apart, ideally the first 3 are 24 hours apart. Try to do one every day for 5 days as your first run. After that 2-3 are good (which is what I do every year or so, just to keep things in perfect shape).

2) Help the process by eating as light as possible during this time. If the first 20 minutes of each treatment is spent draining out the past few days of food, then you're not working on the deeper, hardened layers. You're wasting half the treatment. This isn't like hosing a steel pipe, you have layers of crud in your colon, and even after 5 treatments, you won't have removed everything.

I do an all-juice and smoothie diet 3 days before I start, and stay on just juice for the 2-3 days of treatment. *Great for getting into beach-bod shape too ;)*

3) Try to do this when you can relax afterward. I knew someone who did them on lunch breaks and went back to work, then to the gym. That's better than nothing, but unimaginable for me. Ideally, you go home and relax as your body re-settles, and prepare for a fantastic night of sleep (which almost everyone experiences after colonics).

I'm obviously pro-colonic. I've seen miracles with it in so many people (totally unrelated to CD). Lifetime headaches and migraines gone in 3 days. Focus issues cleared immediately. Insomnia gone overnight. Skin issues cleared in weeks. Most people feel mentally clear immediately, which was my first experience. At the time, I had no health issues I knew of, and I still felt this huge transformation. Clarity that I can't quite express in words, and I got the best night of sleep I had ever had in my entire life. That was it, I was convinced of the powers of hydrotherapy from day one.

The list of effects and benefits is too long to list. Just be sure you do it right, with a qualified person. The good ones will massage exact points through almost the whole session, getting lodged particles to move along. Some have massagers that cover your entire ab area, so the vibration helps dislodge things. Both good.

Done right, colonics will change your very being. You're literally turning a glass of mud into clear water, and your brain will feel it instantly.

And this concludes the sexy topic of colonics :)

How to Beat the Dark Stats

Every time I ask this question, I get resistance. Well, it needs to be asked: Why do 30-55% of people with Celiac (who are GF) never get well and suffer the same premature illness and mortality as those who aren't diagnosed/GF[331]???

Put the Eckhart Tolle book down, I don't need inspired reading or a sunshine enema, I'm not being negative. I'm protecting my fellow Celiac and want to know where all these people are going wrong so we can correct it. I want everyone to be healthy, happy, and live with Joie de Vivre to the end.

"Strict gluten-free diet is mandatory for CD, but it frequently does not lead to normalization of..."[332] [referring to the damage of the intestines]

Why not??? Why are those guts not healing if the person is GF? We can break it down even further:

"After at least 2 years on a strict GFD

-Intestinal damage was completely corrected in only 43.6%

-Intestinal damage was modest in 32.6%

-Intestinal damage was severe in 23.8%"[333]

Two years strict GF and intestinal damage has not healed in 55%? Why?

"After an average of 12 years on a GFD, 31% of patients still have increased inflammation in their intestines."[334]

12 years GF and 31% still show inflammation in their gut (remember that most people will suffer brain damage with no gut damage, which means it's much *much* much *much* worse than 31%). These are all different studies, all consistently showing grim stats. Clearly, we're missing something.

...Now don't get me wrong, I'm not saying it's hopeless. If it was, I wouldn't bother writing this book, I'd be getting my butt bruised learning how to surf. I'm saying we're missing a piece of the puzzle and need to take a "No Celiac Left Behind" approach.

Plenty of studies that follow newly diagnosed patients, even test their brain fog and cognitive function upon diagnosis, then test again at intervals after the patient is gluten-free, show cognitive improvement[335] and even total reversal. Even brains tested after meditation retreats show improvement, but those aren't glutened brains with plaque so hardened you couldn't crack it with a bulldozer. This is a good time to explain what that means. Let's go from guts to brain for a quick minute, so you'll know what happens after gut becomes exhausted...

BRAIN PLAQUE

Called Amyloid Plaque. Amyloid itself is a protein that's deposited everywhere: Brain, liver, kidneys, spleen. Genetically, only 2% of people are susceptible to this, causing dementia, most often Alzheimer's. The other 98% are forming amyloid from environmental factors (food and other toxins, including gluten). Like glycation, you can't un-harden plaque. It suffocates your cells.

Plaque isn't the enemy, it's your well-intentioned friend (with benefits that are back-firing). When you glutenize your brain, it will defend itself any way it can. One of those ways is by forming plaque. In self-defense, it's putting a protective shield around cells and in the process, "freezing" your brain. If that plaque stays there long enough and hardens, your brain mysteriously stops functioning. *It's not that mysterious.* Stop sending toxins to your brain, and plaque can go back to its permanent vacation, where it belongs. It doesn't want to be there, it wants to be in Cancun sipping piña coladas. Amyloid Plaque are like firemen, distant as long as you don't start a fire.

Everyone else is saying "Just go GF and you'll heal, here's a muffin recipe using corn flour and sugar, life is wonderful, glass is half full".

I'm saying "Far too many people aren't healing, make sure you're not one of them. Make sure it's not just your symptoms that are gone, make sure antibodies and all war debris are properly cleaned up, it sometimes takes more than a GF muffin to get to wellness after coming out of a war zone".

Please Keep Reading... Learn it once, it'll serve you forever and beyond gluten...

AMYLOID AND OTHER "FORCED" LINES OF DEFENSE

Amyloid plaque is a good example of what a second line of defense is. First line is supposed to be the blood/brain barrier. But humans, we're *so* smart, we figured out ways to manufacture food that can bypass Nature and break through that barrier. We need to get a little less smart and go back to foods that don't mess with Nature (we're outgunned).

My goal isn't to geek you out or upset you, it's to prevent dementia. Here's why I explain so much detail: When people think they can drink lemon water for a few days and make anything go away, they're more inclined to regularly eat toxic junk. When they're informed and understand that excessive toxins force the body to start forming plaque that has the potential to irreversibly kill their brain function, and simple detox won't clean it up, that piece of cake doesn't look so appealing anymore.

Understanding this not-so-fun concept can help you make better decisions long term. You'll find yourself saying "No, it's not worth it. I'm not eating that junk, I'll just wait until I can get my hands on a healthy version" ...and that decision is one less assault to your system. They add up. This applies to all toxins, not just gluten.

EXTENDED DETOX PROTOCOLS MIGHT BE NEEDED

Brain damage can (usually) be reversed, even with conditions as serious as Alzheimer's and Down's: "Our case report shows that, before concluding in Alzheimer-type dementia in Down's syndrome, a biological search for coeliac disease is useful since a gluten-free diet may improve the psychiatric symptoms."[336]

Symptoms usually improve, but it's important to test and get a clean bill of health. Some elements, like plaque, metals (particularly mercury in the brain... solution to this in the supplements section), mucous in the gut and/or lungs (yes, lungs, caused by gluten/dairy), ...if any of these are still present, the person needs to work with a knowledgeable practitioner and engage in a 12-month customized detox protocol, then re-test.

Think of how long the average detox plan is. 7-21 days, right? *If* that. *"Drink a little nettle tea and you're set."* Oh no, you're not. This is one of the reasons it's important to work with someone who is immersed in gluten because just like regular nutrition doesn't cover gluten well, neither does regular detox. All things gluten are an animal of their own.

227

THE MEDICAL AND LEGAL FACTOR CONTRIBUTE TO THE GRIM STATS

Part of the problem is people knowingly cheat, not yet accepting potential consequences. The bigger problem is people following laws based on a medical and legal system that doesn't yet protect them. With stats like half stay sick, it's time to re-evaluate what we classify as gluten-free.

You have to understand how unregulated the world of gluten-free is. How many packages do you see in stores that say "gluten-free oats"? You see that on the front label to appease your worry about cross-contamination. Who is testing and questioning the contents of that box? So, a Celiac replaces their regular cereal with oatmeal, thinking they're GF, and the antibodies flooding their brain from that oatmeal will eventually cause illness.

Remember the study showing 44% of Celiacs reacting to corn? Well guess what most Celiacs are eating every day in processed foods? 44% reacting... and what? 30-55% of guts don't heal... I don't want to draw unproven conclusions, but would you say at least some of those people aren't getting well due to corn, oats, and whatever else they shouldn't be eating? They should at least be warned there's a risk and be allowed to make their own decision. Well, here it is, you've been warned.

An important takeaway here is that you can't wait for the system to keep you safe. The system is slow, and you don't have that kind of time. This is both scary and overwhelming for most people. Celiac is complicated enough, now we can't trust foods labeled GF? I do understand, and I wish I had a magic wand to fix the system.

3 STEP CHECKLIST

STEP 1: Stop poisoning yourself. You do that by making sure you're 100% gluten free, not just legally gluten free. You'll never get to wellness unless you stop eating the things that are triggering sickness.

STEP 2: Repair. "Modulation of Gut Microbiota-Brain Axis by Probiotics, Prebiotics, and Diet."[337] Sometimes it's as easy as probiotics, sometimes you need cell-renewing strategies. Suggestions are listed in the Supplements chapter, but I advise you to work with a qualified practitioner if possible. Find someone as OCD as me, and someone immersed in the world of gluten (who's not getting their info from flawed Internet articles).

STEP 3: Test for Antibodies. I suggest yearly testing, or at least every other year. It's the only way to keep your eye on things. Antibodies = something is slipping through the cracks and you need to evaluate what you're eating. By monitoring your blood, you can get ahead of damage and take steps to course-correct. If you already do an annual physical, just find a doctor that'll tick off a few extra boxes on the blood work (additional tips in the Testing section).

CURES

A lot of drugs are about to hit the market that "cure" Celiac Disease and allow the person to eat anything they want. The way these drugs work: They turn off the immune response. They turn OFF your immune system.

They turn your immune system, your defense system, OFF.

Let me say it another way: They shut down your immune system and leave you susceptible to every disease known and unknown to man. You're retiring your army, then going into war naked and unarmed. Daily. I can't believe it's legal to even experiment with shutting down a person's immune system, but of cour$e it i$. I promise the Marketing Masters will get called in to figure out how to make this acceptable, probably pitch that it's only the reaction to gluten they're turning off, and the devil only knows what else they'll come up with.

My tiny voice is barely audible against trillion-dollar companies with billion-dollar marketing budgets, so I'll say my peace on this page and leave it to your good judgment when the avalanche of marketing is soon unleashed.

Here's why there's no cure for gluten sensitivity and there will never be: The human body was never designed to eat gluten and we're not smart enough to re-design the human body.

DIGESTIVE ENZYMES

Think Primal: If you need pills to digest something, you probably weren't meant to be eating it.

A company that wanted me to be a brand ambassador for them gave me a sample of their product, just before it hit market. This was first geared for when you get contaminated and meant to help you digest the unintentional consumption of gluten. The way they're selling it is: Take it every time you eat out, just in case. That's brilliant strategy. Guaranteed sales whether the product is needed or not. Genius, actually. We're all scared of being contaminated, why not sell an insurance policy.

I held on to the bottle until I got accidentally contaminated, then took it. Yes, it did something. It prevented me from vomiting, but I felt like I had a cement block in my stomach for a week, with a whole new kind of pain. It wasn't Mike Tyson punching me from the outside, it was his demon double punching me from the inside, with a little less intensity. Migraine for weeks was unchanged. I would have preferred to vomit and be sick the first night rather than feel sick a whole week, constantly wanting to vomit but unable to. It kept coming up, but no matter what I did, couldn't purge. It was disgusting. I could smell and taste it for a week instead of getting it over with in one night.

...Now that's just my personal experience, not a major study with a few thousand people (which the makers of that product, or any of those products, haven't done either). But I'm a good tester because of how acutely I react. Someone who doesn't outwardly show the symptoms as much isn't a good tester because the damage goes undetected. But we know from close examination in studies that the same damage and long-term risks are happening to both those bodies.

WHEN I'M GOOD WITH ENZYMES

I'm good with enzymes if the person's system is devastated and they need to rebuild. The same way probiotics can help rebuild a better colony of inhabitants in your gut, so can enzymes, they can help you process correctly again. But you do this with a qualified practitioner and stop doing it once you've achieved homeostasis. Your body shouldn't need lifelong assistance to eat food. If it does, either you're eating the wrong food, or something in your body needs healing. Does that make natural sense to you?

I don't recommend pills to help digest food, nor deal with contamination. If you're contaminated, don't block or suppress it, let your body do its job. Help your body in natural ways, like lemon water or activated charcoal, but don't stop the engine.

CELIAC DISEASE IS COMPLEX

I should publish an entire book using only titles of studies, what an interesting story they would tell all on their own...

"Celiac disease: how complicated can it get?"[338]

While that one is talking more about genes, t-cells, and peptides... and complicated as the biological elements are, so are the psychological aspects. From documented denial and outright refusal to testing[339], to how the news is taken, if ever diagnosed...

DID THEY SAY "TAKE TIME TO GRIEVE"?!?

Being diagnosed with any disorder isn't good news, but Celiac Disease causes somewhat different emotional difficulty. The world doesn't reject you when you have cancer. The world doesn't reject you, even with other disorders that affect diet, like diabetes or Crohn's. We don't mock people with diabetes, we sympathize with them. Yet we hang gluten-free people out to dry, mock, shame, ridicule... it's worse than schoolyard bullying.

And it's becoming weaved into culture. That's a dangerous thing. I saw a movie where the star is chatting with the love interest. She's casually talking about herself and builds in: "I'm calling bullshit on anyone who suddenly develops an allergy to gluten in the last 6 years". Can you imagine them mocking cancer in a movie? Pink running shoes would hit the streets in protests everywhere telling the world to boycott the movie. Somebody would get their head chopped off and the producers would issue a public apology. *And it wouldn't happen again.*

Alton Brown, Food Network Star, September 16, 2016, in The New York Times (did that get a few eyes?) promoting his new book: "Unless you have a medical bracelet that says celiac, shut up and eat the food." *Nice.* Thanks for your input Alton. ...And where are the lovely Celiac Associations in all this??? Busy printing their next set of "1 in 133" t-shirts.

I won't digress here, but it's such an important element, I dedicated a whole module to it in my course. Health Coaches need to understand what their clients are facing, and doctors need to understand the reluctance to testing. All of the above need to understand the TLC needed after diagnoses.

Many countries have done studies and found consistent results: People diagnosed with Celiac feel like an outcast from the rest of society and they feel a part of themselves has died.

For most people, it's not about simple diet changes. It's about being different from everyone else. It's like being voted off the island. Happy Hour after work, when everyone else is munching on anything they want, isn't so happy for a Celiac. Teenager? Multiply that feeling by a thousand. Pizza is as much a part of school as the books themselves. Cookie break starts in daycare and never ends… we still have cookies and muffins at executive board meetings (all that's missing is the glass of milk, but I'm sure the Dairy Association is working on it).

Canada has done more than one study, finding frustration and isolation high. "Eating shifted from the public to the domestic sphere and there were feelings of social isolation."[340]
Their conclusion on another study: "need to improve the training and education of dietitians, other health providers and the food service industry workers about coeliac disease and a gluten-free diet."[341] Sadly, most of those dietitians and health providers are all over the web, talking about how gluten isn't so bad.

Over to the UK: "elevated levels of psychological distress, including depression, anxiety and social phobia… five key categories: living with widespread ignorance; social invisibility; creating a coeliac community; a changed identity; grief - and accepting the trade-off… Grief was experienced in relation to a loss of the former diet, changed personal and social identities, loss of social confidence and loss of social activities."[342]

The word "grief", I've seen it in multiple Celiac studies. The first time I saw it wasn't in a study, but in the Canadian Celiac Association's Guide. They suggested a newly diagnosed person should take the time to grieve and then they proceeded to give negligent advice (like ice-cream being safe, with no breakdown of ingredients, meanwhile, 95% of grocery store ice cream has gluten in it). I wasn't very kind to them then, and I'm not now, for even more reasons. I don't say this to vent. I want to show how much support every Celiac is lacking and how even the main national associations are leading them wrong. I wonder if it's a coincidence that the authors of "The Coeliac Syndrome"[343] from 1948 were guys named Grieve and Pitt.

233

PURE GF IS DECADENCE

When I used to do house calls and kitchen makeovers, I'd always go over with a raw cheesecake (usually a flavor I already knew they loved from their food diary and my initial questionnaire).

"How are you today? Why don't you make us some tea to go along with our raw salted caramel cheesecake while we review a few things?"

After the first bite: "OMG this is the best cheesecake I've eaten in my entire life!!! Will I get to eat like this gluten-free?"

"Yes, and better, I was crunched on time and rushed a bit. By the way, it's not just gluten free, it's dairy and sugar free too."

In my mind I would think *"What the hell are those fools doing over there, telling people to grieve, as if they died"*. And that's right in their welcome guide! What a way for someone to be introduced to their new lifestyle instead of with a decadent cake.

POWER TIP TO HEALTH COACHES: Before you rip apart someone's kitchen and throw 90% of their food into garbage bags, start the session off with a decadent food and they won't feel so doomed.

My raw cheesecakes and truffles are still the unrivaled favorites at any party I go to. People actually text to find out when I'm arriving because they know they better be there before me, since no matter how much food I bring, it's all gone within 15 minutes. I'm not even a sweets person, I'm stronger on savory.

Did someone say "deprived"? Try "coveted" and people begging me on hands and knees to make them my gluten-free, dairy-free, sugar-free, toxin-free luscious food. *I'm starting to wonder if I should be opening a GF Bistro.*

NO GRIEVING. It's a time to celebrate the re-discovery of awesome, flavor-rich, powerful, nutritious, real food. **Celiac Disease is a wakeup call, not a death sentence.**

5. Testing

I'm going to start with tips on this one because they're as important as the tests themselves and information you should know *before* scheduling tests.

POWER TIPS

1) CHOOSING YOUR PRACTITIONER. Ideally, you're working with a holistic or functional medicine doctor who makes it their business to stay up to date. I've met dinosaur MD's whose last formal training, *for anything*, was 1978. They did their 8 years of schooling and they're not interested in more. The only updates they get is from pharmaceutical reps (salespeople, not medical people), on what newest drugs to prescribe. Stay away from the dinosaurs so that you don't perish like the dinosaurs did.

If it's a doctor you've had for a long time, it can feel disarming, I completely understand. But if they're not doing right by you, please find the courage and do what you know you need to do.

I'm not bashing all doctors, there are many good ones. The last one I saw was incredibly nice and completely informed. Solved my mystery in one visit and had initial test results in my hands in one day.

2) GET YOUR RESULTS. Before booking your appointment for any tests (including nutritional deficiencies), I advise you to ensure that you will get a copy of your results. I've had doctor's offices tell me they don't do that... perfect, thanks, spared me getting tested all over again elsewhere. I call another clinic.

The point isn't to turn into your own pathologist, but when it comes to basic "within norm" levels, you don't need a medical degree to see that you're dangerously low. Example: Normal Vitamin D level is 50. If you're at 51, you'll "pass" your doctor's test and he'll tell you that you're fine, and today you might be. Two weeks from now you start falling below 50. It's not like you're going to run blood tests every month, so pay attention when you're borderline on anything and power up. Doctor's offices are very black and white with positive/negative, but it's never that simple.

You don't want to be borderline. You want to be optimal. You want some buffer space. 50% of heart attack patients are in "normal range" on yearly visits. Something is wrong with those numbers.

RDA's were established in the 1940's and levels haven't been adjusted since. Things have changed, *just a little,* since the 1940's when the Recommended Daily Allowances were set. The medical system and government systems are Dead Halt Slow. If they were ship captains, we'd all drown. Actually, we *are* drowning, we're in a global health crisis that no other generation or time could have ever imagined.

3) NEWLY DIAGNOSED, DON'T TEST FOR FOOD INTOLERANCE (YET). It's an expensive, useless exercise. I'll save you money: You're allergic to a hundred foods. ...Let me explain: When your system is a disaster (which is where most newly diagnosed people are), you'll test positive for a lot of allergies which will all quickly reverse when you become gluten-free. I spent $2,000 to find out I was allergic to 125 foods, including lettuce and tomatoes, only to find out it was all false and 60 days after being GF, 120 of the 125 were fine again. The 5 that remained: wheat and its cousins. If you want to test with accuracy, do it 6-12 months after you've been strictly gluten-free.

By the way, I ran that expensive test with the same doctor that first realized my symptoms might be coming from gluten. So, while he knew enough to test for Celiac, he didn't know enough to tell me to wait a while before testing for other food intolerances. I'm *not* complaining, the man was a godsend. He'll always be a good guy in my eyes, he solved the mystery. I'm just pointing out that you have to remain as knowledgeable as possible and always stay in the driver's seat with this thing, because Celiac Disease is a detailed disease and instincts don't always serve well...

...When someone finds out they got severely sick from a food, it's a natural instinctive reaction to then want to find out what else they might be reacting to. But in this case, it's better to wait, and it takes experience to know that. Now you know.

ALWAYS WORK WITH A PHYSICIAN WITH ACCESS TO TESTS

Always coordinate with a physician. When I suggest taking control of one's health, it's never ever in a Wild Wild West scenario. I didn't do that with my own health, I went to the people who had access to testing machines (I just wasn't afraid to fire the ones who didn't seem like they were up to date).

Taking control means being informed and making sure all relevant up-to-date tests that are available are being applied. There might also be other underlying issues that require attention, and that's something a standard health coach or even naturopathic doctor can't help you with. Statistically, someone with one autoimmune issue will develop 2-3 other issues (that's what happens when your system is compromised, and why pills that shut off your system to allow you to eat gluten are a very bad idea).

Work with a physician, just make sure your voice isn't lost and they're working to help you find the root cause of things. Their goal should be to bring you back to your natural healthy state, drug-free.

TIP TO MY FELLOW CANADIANS: You wouldn't believe how much more doctors "care" and pay attention when you pay for their time. You get what you pay for and even though we're taxed higher than Mafia loans and technically pay for it, Medicare is a very different world from private. If you can afford it, it's worth it and can spare you a lot of time and pain. I went through 6 doctors (not counting several in the E.R.) and all I ended up with was being 10 seconds away from organ failure and being told it's time to see a psychiatrist. If I think about the 15 or so doctors I saw between the ones I went to and the random ones in the E.R., the only words I can think of are: "Negligent, ignorant, inhuman." One told me it's common for unmarried women my age (38 at the time) to go through a crisis. ?!@$?$?^#%?^$?% I thought I time-travelled back to 1960 and then realized I hadn't been born yet then. *I feel for the women that came before us.*

I paid for a doctor to listen and everything got solved in 15 minutes. ...Though in all fairness, he was kinder than he needed to be, I don't think it was only my Amex.

Testing Methods

1) **BLOOD** (Need to still be eating gluten)

A) Transglutaminase (autoimmune response, suggesting Celiac)

B) Endomysium (autoimmune response, suggesting Celiac)

C) Gluten Peptides (good, depending on how many being tested, usually it's only one peptide, #33, and that's present in only 50% of cases)

D) Gliadin & Deaminated Gliadin (Testing wheat allergy, not Celiac. Allergy can be outgrown, Celiac is irreversible once triggered.)

While antibodies are a better bet (because you don't have the same hit & miss as with biopsy swab... blood is evenly affected), the levels of antibodies generally correlate with intestinal damage. On average, blood tests will come back positive in only 31% of cases until further damage is done[344]. In stages 1 and 2 of damage, the result often comes back false negative[345]. The "fail" line isn't set high enough yet within the medical system.

However, there is one combination of testing that has apparently been accurate, and don't play mad scientists here, you're not expected to understand this... just take it with you to your doctor and ask them to test for this specific combination: "IgA + IgG a-DGP plus a-tTG had 100% positive and negative predictive values."[346]

...Now you know what I meant in the beginning of this book when I said nothing about gluten is clear cut.

The European protocol for blood testing: "Sensitivity, specificity, positive, and negative predictive value of QUANTA Flash h-tTG IgA were excellent. The cut-off providing an optimized PPV for histological lesions compatible for celiac disease (Marsh ≥2) for the QUANTA Flash h-tTG IgA is 350 CU (15×) in adult and 560 CU (28×) in children."[347]

POWER TIP: You might also want to ask for one more thing. CRP (C-Reactive Protein) is a marker for system inflammation. You're getting a needle in your arm, might as well make it count and get a full diagnostic.

2) BIOPSY (If you've been GF a while, intestines may have healed and show false results. Healing can be as fast as 2-3 weeks, so if you started out with an elimination diet, biopsy will often give false results)

Remember the flaws regarding biopsy. The more damaged you are, the more accurate biopsy will be. This is still the only way to get an official letter from your doctor's office confirming you have Celiac Disease. The one useful function of having that letter is that in some countries (yes for Canada & U.S., check with yours), a confirmed Celiac gets a tax break in the difference of cost for GF food. You'll need to submit that letter with your taxes the first time you declare, and after that it'll be on file.

The way to do this is a bit tedious. You keep all your food receipts and one by one indicate difference in price. So if you spend $6.99 on a loaf of GF bread, and standard bread is $1.99, you get some amount of tax break on the difference of $5.00. If you have a large family and plan to buy a lot of packaged GF food, it can make a difference.

3) GENE TEST (Do not need to be eating gluten)

Usually a very simple saliva swab. We used to think gene testing was 100% accurate and that you absolutely had to have one of two genes, HLA-DQ2 or HLA-DQ8, to fall into the Celiac category.

However, a newer study showed that neither of these genes were present in 7% of their biopsy confirmed Celiac subjects, and another study had 5% missing the genes.

This means gene testing is not absolute, but only 93% or so accurate with the stats we have to date. Still quite accurate compared to everything else, and the least invasive. It also doesn't rely on level of damage, it just tells you if you're susceptible to CD specifically or not. It doesn't tell you if you're reacting with NCGS.

4) STOOL TEST (Need to still be eating gluten)

I'm giving you all possible options but will tell you I don't suggest stool test for gluten. There are too many variables that fluctuate here. They'll test for gliadin and transglutaminase antibodies, which you'll get better results with on a blood test. I prefer stool testing for gut status rather than reaction to gluten.

5) ELIMINATION TEST

By far the most popular. Costs nothing, no doctor needed, you get off gluten and see if you feel better, then get back on and see if you react. It works well if done right.

COMMON PITFALLS OF THE ELIMINATION TEST:

A) You don't do it long enough. Gluten antibodies can stay in your system 3-6 months. I've never known anyone to be 100% strictly gluten free for that long unless they know they have to be. Most people try a few days, maybe a week, then go back to regular food habits.

B) You eat out and can't be positive of food safety. Again, I've never known a soul who will abruptly never eat a bite out for 3-6 months to do an elimination test. But all it takes is 10mg (0.002 teaspoon) to get a reaction and keep it going for weeks. That's literally a drop of contamination, just from a waiter touching your plate after touching a bread basket.

C) You don't have an accurate list and are eating foods you think are GF, but they're not. Since the symptoms don't go away, "oh, it must not have been gluten then". Remember that legally gluten free doesn't mean it's actually gluten free (if you haven't already, read Bonus "20 PPM's").

STAY IN THE DRIVER'S SEAT

This is just to make a simple point of why it's important for you to stay in the driver's seat... This paper is discussing the Marsh Method/biopsy: "We believe that a simplification of the current histological classifications of CD is necessary to make the work of pathologists more uniform and to facilitate the relationship between pathologists and clinicians."[348] ...Thanks Guys. We certainly wouldn't want to inconvenience pathologists or clinicians. Let's make things "more uniform". I have no idea how that math works since no two Celiacs will ever be exactly the same. And why *have* pathologists if they're not closely studying each individual? Isn't that the reason for their existence? Why not replace them with robots and software? It's an honest question.

Until the world acknowledges that CD affects more than 1%, that gluten is disrupting everyone's gut, and that a major cause of brain and systemic damage is coming from grains, the medical world is not going to pay the attention you need. You have the knowledge now (seriously, you rock for reading this whole book), so be sure to maintain control of your health.

Testing is Misrepresenting How Many Affected

I've put a spotlight on the monumental room for error with biopsy, even the system knows how flawed biopsy is, in 2006 the Journal of Gastroenterology said biopsy isn't the gold standard because they know most people are slipping through the cracks: "Conventional histology is not anymore a gold standard in the diagnosis. The diagnostic criteria need thus to be revised."[349] ...Over a decade later, biopsy is still the only way to be diagnosed, nothing has been revised.

Side Note: The exact same year that the American Journal of Gastroenterology said biopsy is not the gold standard anymore, another study (smaller, Family Medicine, University of NC) starts off its study with: "biopsy is the gold standard for diagnosing celiac disease."[350] Then they proceed to provide 4 types of blood tests to "serve as a first-step diagnostic tool to identify biopsy candidates". I don't point this out to criticize, just the opposite. I want to point out that the topic is a mess, and I can understand why most doctors are misinformed. Even the ones taking some time out to read actual studies are facing hit & miss, depending on which article they happen to read.

You can't wrap your mind around this topic until after you've read 500+ studies and start connecting dots, seeing flaws, seeing how gray data can fuzz the conclusions, ... I'm convinced you can't master this topic without giving it exclusive dedication for a significant period of time. There's just no other way around sorting through so much conflicting information.

BLOOD TESTS MAKING THEIR WAY THROUGH THE SYSTEM

One group of doctors put out a plea for blood tests right in the title of their study: "Selective immunoglobulin A deficiency and celiac disease: let's give serology a chance."[351] I might be the only person on earth who read that study.

Gluten damage was determined via biopsy 6 decades ago, so they stuck to it: "abnormalities of the lining of the small intestine were demonstrated beyond doubt by Paulley in 1954."[352] ...But there have been some updates since 1954, most importantly: To not wait for total devastation, a.k.a. Total Villous Atrophy, the same way we don't wait for stage 4 cancer before acting.

Blood tests are usually better than biopsy, certainly less invasive, however, to be clear, blood tests aren't perfect either and there's room for error there too. I won't get into all of it (I want to cure your insomnia, but not like this), but I will tell you the system is well aware of the gaps: "Recent literature data showed that serology... seems to be ineffective in detecting most of the patients affected by subclinical/silent disease[353]"... meaning it can miss early stages because the blood isn't poisoned enough yet.

Unless you're at stage 4, the data says that blood tests will be incorrect 69% of the time.[354]

I've given you a checklist of tests that give you the best odds for accuracy and how you can beat these numbers, with the most updated information we have. The question is, do you even want to bother with testing after reading this book?

THERE ARE NO ABSOLUTES IN THE WORLD OF GLUTEN

It's a complex spider web, some rings are perfectly woven, others have gaps, it's a work in progress. Our generation won't be here to see it in any exact form.

However, with all the tools we have, we could do a lot better. Better yet, since we know gluten is causing all this chaos, why don't we stop trying to figure out how to force ourselves to digest it and just stop eating it. Genetically Modified Wheat for Celiacs? *Seriously?*

If I had known all this information years ago, Celiac or not, I would have immediately stopped eating gluten. Why would I invite trouble into my body and brain? It's a dance with the devil that we could all do without.

The snail-paced progress of the system is costing millions of lives. In the 1960's (not that long ago in medical terms), they were still blaming mothers for Celiac and accusing them of neglecting their children. That's not a folk tale, it's in the actual medical documentation, look at the title of this study: (1964) "Neglected Children and the Celiac Syndrome."[355]

Mothers were being accused of neglecting their children, meanwhile the cause for their kids' decline in health was coming from feeding them the "healthy grains" the government was telling the public to eat 4 servings of a day at that time. Today it's "healthy whole grains" and more of it. "My Plate" issued by the USDA for 2015-2020 suggests a quarter of your food intake should be grains, and don't forget the dairy[356]. Zero mention of organic anything.

European Testing Modified to Antibodies in 2012

2001, ANTIBODIES IGNORED

Amsterdam, 2001, United European Gastroenterology Week: "The finding of circulating antibodies . . . supports the diagnosis but is not essential, and should not be used for diagnosis without histologic confirmation."[359] [histologic = tissue damage, they're referring to biopsy].

"The finding of circulating antibodies is not essential" ...that's what your gastroenterologist was being taught (still is in most places).

I don't care about water under the bridge, the point being made here is it's a work in progress and they're still being taught things today that will look very different in a decade or two.

2012, ANTIBODIES BECOME MAIN METHOD TO TEST FOR CHILDREN

The European Society for Pediatric Gastroenterology Hepatology and Nutrition (ESPGHAN) feel they have enough accuracy to predict Marsh levels 2 and higher. In a 2018 study, they took kids considered high risk for Celiac (diabetes and/or Celiac relatives) and tested for antibodies. Every kid with high levels of antibodies tested positive for Celiac on biopsy. And it's important to note they were all asymptomatic. "This study provides further evidence that the guidelines for diagnosing CD by the serology-based pathway should be extended to these children."[360]

GERMANY

This was studied again in Germany: "...we validated the TTG-IgA procedure and the TTG-DGL procedure in identification of pediatric patients with or without celiac disease, without biopsy."[361]

SWEDEN

"Celiac disease can be associated with severe neurological symptoms...a wide spectrum of neurological and psychiatric symptoms (cerebellar ataxia, neuromuscular manifestations, epilepsy, dementia)... Analysis of gliadin antibodies should be considered in suspected cases."[362]

245

18 COUNTRIES COLLABORATE

Now with 63 collaborators from various cities in Germany, Spain, France, UK, Hungary, Finland, Romania, Italy, Greece, Denmark, Netherlands, Iran, Slovenia, Austria, Belgium, Czech Republic, Israel, and Portugal (Canada and U.S. nowhere in sight), and it's encouraging to see a title like "Accuracy in Diagnosis of Celiac Disease Without Biopsies in Clinical Practice."

Their conclusion: "Children can be accurately diagnosed with celiac disease without biopsy analysis. Diagnosis based on level of TGA-IgA 10-fold or more the ULN, a positive result from the EMA tests in a second blood sample, and the presence of at least 1 symptom could avoid risks and costs of endoscopy for more than half the children with celiac disease worldwide."[363] I'm looking forward to adults getting the same privilege.

The Italians are calling it "the 'biopsy-sparing' protocol."[364]

It's quite possible some doctors in North America have started working more with blood tests/antibodies rather than biopsy, though I haven't heard much splash about it, nor have I seen a lot of papers. Canada reviewed the European findings: "The TTG is a very sensitive screen for CD, but positive predictive value improves with a positive EMA titer"[365], but they haven't changed policy yet.

I'd obviously like to see us do away with all of this and just return to real no-risk food, but at least there's an inch of progress here. Just remember:
1) This is detecting level 2 and higher
2) Still not 100% accurate
3) You can still sustain damage at levels 0 and 1

GEEK TALK (use this for blood testing)

If you're a doctor or wish to take this to yours: "Sensitivity, specificity, positive, and negative predictive value of QUANTA Flash h-tTG IgA were excellent. The cut-off providing an optimized PPV for histological lesions compatible for celiac disease (Marsh ≥2) for the QUANTA Flash h-tTG IgA is 350 CU (15×) in adult and 560 CU (28×) in children."[366]

This officially concludes all parts of this book. I wish you Love, Laughter, Health to your last breath.
    -Jaqui

REFERENCES

[1] Lionetti E, Leonardi S, et al. Gluten Psychosis: Confirmation of a New Clinical Entity. Nutrients. 2015 Jul 8;7(7):5532-9. doi: 10.3390/nu7075235. PubMed PMID: 26184290; PubMed Central PMCID: PMC4517012.

[2] Cohen N. M. (1987) "The significance of long-term changes in human diet and food economy," in Food and Evolution: Toward a Theory of Human Food Habits, eds Harris M., Ross E. B., editors. (Philadelphia: Temple University Press;), 261-284.

[3] BMJ, Vol.318, June 26, 1999

[4] Paola Bressan and Peter Kramer. "Bread and Other Edible Agents of Mental Disease" Front Hum Neurosci. 2016; 10: 130. Published online 2016 Mar 29. doi:10.3389/fnhum.2016.00130

[5] Dr. Fasano, MD, Pediatric Gastroenterologist, Founder/Director of the Center for Celiac Research at Massachusetts General Hospital

[6] R Ciccocioppo, A Di Sabatino, and G R Corazza. "The immune recognition of gluten in coeliac disease" Clin Exp Immunol. 2005 Jun; 140(3): 408-416. doi: 10.1111/j.1365-2249.2005.02783.x

[7] The University of Chicago Celiac Disease Center, Impact, Vol 7, Issue 3, 2007

[8] Jabri B, Sollid LM. T Cells in Celiac Disease. J Immunol. 2017 Apr 15;198(8):3005-3014. doi: 10.4049/jimmunol.1601693. Review. PubMed PMID: 28373482; PubMed Central PMCID: PMC5426360.

[9] Fabris M, Visentini D, De Re V, Picierno A, Maieron R, Cannizzaro R, Villalta D, Curcio F, De Vita S, Tonutti E. Elevated B cell-activating factor of the tumour necrosis factor family in coeliac disease. Scand J Gastroenterol. 2007 Dec;42(12):1434-9. PubMed PMID: 17852877.

[10] BMJ 2017;357:j1892

[11] Epidemiology: May 2017 - Volume 28 - Issue 3 - p e24-e25 doi: 10.1097/EDE.0000000000000640

[12] Dufault R, Schnoll R, Lukiw WJ, Leblanc B, Cornett C, Patrick L, Wallinga D, Gilbert SG, Crider R. Mercury exposure, nutritional deficiencies and metabolic disruptions may affect learning in children. Behav Brain Funct. 2009 Oct 27;5:44. doi: 10.1186/1744-9081-5-44. Erratum in: Behav Brain Funct. 2018 Feb 7;14 (1):3. PubMed PMID: 19860886; PubMed Central PMCID: PMC2773803.

[13] "Oral manifestations of celiac disease: a clinical guide for dentists" J Mich Dent Assoc. 2011 Oct;93(10):42-6.PMID: 22073722

[14] "Dental and Oral Considerations in Pediatric Celiac Disease." Journal of Dentistry Child (Chic). 2016;83(2):67-70. PMID: 27620516

[15] FDA, U.S. Department of Health, Food, Guidance and Regulation, Guidance Documents & Regulatory Information by Topic, Chemical Contaminants, Metals, Natural Toxins & Pesticides: "Guidance for Industry: Action Levels for Poisonous or Deleterious Substances in Human Food and Animal Feed"

[16] Agriculture and Agri-Food Canada 2013, 2012

[17] NPD Group 2013

[18] Ciaccio EJ, Lewis SK, Biviano AB, Iyer V, Garan H, Green PH. Cardiovascular involvement in celiac disease. World J Cardiol. 2017 Aug 26;9(8):652-666. doi: 10.4330/wjc.v9.i8.652. Review. PubMed PMID: 28932354; PubMed Central PMCID: PMC5583538.

[19] On the coeliac affection. St Bart's Hosp Rep. 1888;24:17-20. [For a more recent comment on Gee's paper see Dowd B, Walker-Smith J. Samuel Gee, Aretaeus, and the coeliac affection. Br Med J 1974;2(5909):45-47; and Lewkonia RM and Baker P's subsequent letters in the Brit Med J. 1974;2(5916):442]

[20] Miller R. Two Cases of Cœliac Infantilism in the Convalescent (Non-diarrhœic) Stage. Proc R Soc Med. 1923;16(Sect Study Dis Child):22-4. PubMed PMID: 20907732.

[21] Low GC. DISCUSS ON ON SPRUE AND COELIAC DISEASE. Proc R Soc Med. 1924;17(Sect Trop Dis Parasitol):23-4. Pubmed PMID: 19984098; PubMed Central PMCID: PMC2201294.

[22] Poynton FJ. A Case of Cœliac Disease with Glycosuria. Proc R Soc Med. 1925;18(Sect Study Dis Child):38-40. PubMed PMID: 20909081.

[23] Parsons LG. The Bone Changes Occurring in Renal and Coeliac Infantilism and their Relationship to Rickets: Part II. Coeliac Rickets. Arch Dis Child. 1927;2(10):198-211.21. Pubmed PMID: 21031697; PubMed Central PMCID: PMC1974976.

[24] Miller R. A Note on Gluteal Wasting as a Sign of Cœliac Disease. Arch Dis Child. 1927;2(9):189-90. PubMed PMID: 21031695; PubMed Central PMCID: PMC1974958.

[25] Emslie M. Coeliac Disease. Proc R Soc Med. 1928 Feb;21(4):563-4. PubMed PMID: 19986297; PubMed Central PMCID: PMC2102063.

[26] Little H. Chronic Intestinal Indigestion (Coeliac Disease). Can Med Assoc J. 1929 May;20(5):500-2. PubMed PMID: 20317330; PubMed Central PMCID: PMC1710531.

[27] Parsons LG, Hawksley JC. Studies in the Anæmias of Infancy and Early Childhood: Part III. The anhæmatopoietic anæmias (deficiency diseases of the erythron): nutritional anæmia, and the anæmias of prematurity, scurvy and cœliac disease. Arch Dis Child. 1933 Apr;8(44):117-44. PubMed PMID: 21031916; PubMed Central PMCID: PMC1975260.

[28] Grenet P, de Paillerets F, Gallet JP, Gubert JP, Olivier C. [Anorexic forms of celiac syndromes]. Ann Pediatr (Paris). 1972 Jun-Jul;19(6):491-7. French. PubMed PMID: 4506676.

[29] Mårild K, Størdal K, Bulik CM, et al. Celiac Disease and Anorexia Nervosa: A Nationwide Study. Pediatrics. 2017;139(5):e20164367

[30] Morris JS, Ajdukiewicz AB, Read AE. Neurological disorders and adult coeliac disease. Gut. 1970 Jul;11(7):549-54. PubMed PMID: 4318028; PubMed Central PMCID: PMC1553079.

[31] Vogten AJ, Peña AS. Coeliac disease: one century after Samuel Gee (1888). Neth J Med. 1987 Dec;31(5-6):253-5. PubMed PMID: 3323922.

[32] C. Roberts and K. Manchester, "Dental Disease," in The Archaeology of Disease (New York: Cornell University Press, 2005), 63-83; M. N. Cohen and G. M. M. Crane-Kramer, editors' summation, in Ancient Health: Skeletal Indicators of Agricultural and Economic Intensification (Gainesville: University Press of Florida, 2007), 320-43; L. Cordain, "Cereal Grains: Humanity's Double-Edged Sword," in Evolutionary Aspects of Nutrition and Health, ed. A. P. Simopoulos (Basel: Karger, 1999);84: 19-73.

[33] van den Broeck HC, de Jong HC, Salentijn EM, Dekking L, Bosch D, Hamer RJ, Gilissen LJ, van der Meer IM, Smulders MJ. Presence of celiac disease epitopes in modern and old hexaploid wheat varieties: wheat breeding may have contributed to increased prevalence of celiac disease. Theor Appl

Genet. 2010 Nov;121(8):1527-39. doi: 10.1007/s00122-010-1408-4. Epub 2010 Jul 28. PubMed PMID: 20664999; PubMed Central PMCID: PMC2963738.

[34] Oxilia G, Peresani M, Romandini M, Matteucci C, Spiteri CD, Henry AG, Schulz D, Archer W, Crezzini J, Boschin F, Boscato P, Jaouen K, Dogandzic T, Broglio A, Moggi-Cecchi J, Fiorenza L, Hublin JJ, Kullmer O, Benazzi S. Earliest evidence of dental caries manipulation in the Late Upper Palaeolithic. Sci Rep. 2015 Jul 16;5:12150. doi: 10.1038/srep12150. PubMed PMID: 26179739; PubMed Central PMCID: PMC4504065.

[35] Cohen, Ancient Health, 320-43.

[36] Price, Weston A. Nutrition and Physical Degeneration: A Comparison of Primitive and Modern Diets and Their Effects 1939. Paul B. Hoeber, Inc; Medical Book Department of Harper & Brothers.

[37] Hogerzeil SJ, van Hemert AM, Veling W, Hoek HW. Incidence of schizophrenia among migrants in the Netherlands: a direct comparison of first contact longitudinal register approaches. Soc Psychiatry Psychiatr Epidemiol. 2017 Feb;52(2):147-154. doi: 10.1007/s00127-016-1310-8. Epub 2016 Nov 15. Erratum in: Soc Psychiatry Psychiatr Epidemiol. 2017 Aug 19;:. PubMed PMID: 27847980; PubMed Central PMCID: PMC5329083.

[38] Dickson BC, Streutker CJ, Chetty R. Coeliac disease: an update for pathologists. Journal of Clinical Pathology. 2006;59(10):1008-1016. doi:10.1136/jcp.2005.035345.

[39] J Neurol Neurosurg Psychiatry, 2002;72:560-563

[40] HEPATOLOGY, Vol. 46, No. 5, 2007

[41] Biagi F, Marchese A, Ferretti F, Ciccocioppo R, Schiepatti A, Volta U, Caio G, Ciacci C, Zingone F, D'Odorico A, Carroccio A, Ambrosiano G, Mansueto P, Gasbarrini A, Piscaglia AC, Andrealli A, Astegiano M, Segato S, Neri M, Meggio A, de Pretis G, De Vitis I, Gobbi P, Corazza GR. A multicentre case control study on complicated coeliac disease: two different patterns of natural history, two different prognoses. BMC Gastroenterol. 2014 Aug 7;14:139. doi: 10.1186/1471-230X-14-139. PubMed PMID: 25103857; PubMed Central PMCID: PMC4127435.

[42] Gut 2006;55:1037-1046

[43] Gastroenterology 2001;120:636-651

[44] Gasbarrini G., Ciccocioppo R., et al. Club del Tenue Study Group . (2001)."Coeliac disease in the elderly. A multicentre Italian study". Gerontology 47, 306-310. 10.1159/000052819

[45] NEJM Oct 23, 2003;1673-4

[46] "Genetic Testing" U of Chicago Celiac Disease Center

[47] Ihara M, Makino F, Sawada H, Mezaki T, Mizutani K, Nakase H, Matsui M, Tomimoto H, Shimohama S. Gluten sensitivity in Japanese patients with adult-onset cerebellar ataxia. Intern Med. 2006;45(3):135-40. Epub 2006 Mar 1. PubMed PMID: 16508226.

[48] Datta Gupta S. Pathology of celiac disease: a brief review. Trop Gastroenterol. 2013 Oct-Dec;34(4):207-26. Review. PubMed PMID: 25046883.

[49] Kaukinen K, Partanen J, Mäki M, Collin P. HLA-DQ typing in the diagnosis of celiac disease. Am J Gastroenterol. 2002 Mar;97(3):695-9. PubMed PMID: 11922565.

[50] "Gluten Freedom", Dr. Fasano, pediatric gastroenterologist, world-renowned expert in gluten related disorders, Director of The Celiac Research Center in Maryland

[51] ARCH INTERN MED/Vol 163, Feb 10, 2003

[52] Casella G, Pozzi R, et al. Mood disorders and non-celiac gluten sensitivity. Minerva Gastroenterol Dietol. 2017 Mar;63(1):32-37. doi: 10.23736/S1121-421X.16.02325-4. Epub 2016 Sep 20. Review. PubMed PMID: 27647538.

[53] Jackson JR, Eaton WW, Cascella NG, Fasano A, Kelly DL. Neurologic and Psychiatric Manifestations of Celiac Disease and Gluten Sensitivity. The Psychiatric quarterly. 2012;83(1):91-102. doi:10.1007/s11126-011-9186-y.

[54] JAMA, Sept 16, 2009, Vol 302, No.11

[55] Casella G, Pozzi R, et al. Mood disorders and non-celiac gluten sensitivity. Minerva Gastroenterol Dietol. 2017 Mar;63(1):32-37. doi: 10.23736/S1121-421X.16.02325-4. Epub 2016 Sep 20. Review. PubMed PMID: 27647538

[56] Pennisi, Manuela et al. "Neurophysiology of the 'Celiac Brain': Disentangling Gut-Brain Connections." Frontiers in Neuroscience 11 (2017): 498. PMC. Web. 1 Dec. 2017

[57] Porcelli, Brunetta et al. "Celiac and Non-Celiac Gluten Sensitivity: A Review on the Association with Schizophrenia and Mood Disorders." Auto-Immunity Highlights 5.2 (2014): 55-61. PMC. Web. 1 Dec. 2017

[58] Arshad I, Javeed A, Ullah U. Patient with Gluten Encephalopathy Presenting with Neuropsychiatric Symptoms. Am J Med. 2018 Feb;131(2):e49-e50. doi: 10.1016/j.amjmed.2017.09.023. Epub 2017 Oct 9. PubMed PMID: 29024626.

[59] Poloni N, Vender S, Bolla E, Bortolaso P, Costantini C, Callegari C. Gluten encephalopathy with psychiatric onset: case report. Clin Pract Epidemiol Ment Health. 2009 Jun 26;5:16. doi: 10.1186/1745-0179-5-16. PubMed PMID: 19558661; PubMed Central PMCID: PMC2711951.

[60] National Institutes of Health (U.S. 2012)

[61] Briani C, Zara G, Alaedini A, Grassivaro F, Ruggero S, Toffanin E, et al. Neurological complications of celiac disease and autoimmune mechanisms: A prospective study. Journal of Neuroimmunology. 2008;195:171-175.

[62] Hadjivassiliou M, Grunewald RA, Chattopadhyay AK, Davies-Jones GA, Gibson A, Jarratt JA, et al. Clinical, radiological, neurophysiological, and neuropathological characteristics of gluten ataxia. Lancet. 1998;352:1582-1585.

[63] O'Farrelly C. Is villous atrophy always and only the result of gluten sensitive disease of the intestine? Eur J Gastroenterol Hepatol. 2000 Jun;12(6):605-8. Review. PubMed PMID: 10912475.

[64] Conti V, Leone MC, Casato M, Nicoli M, Granata G, Carlesimo M. High prevalence of gluten sensitivity in a cohort of patients with undifferentiated connective tissue disease. Eur Ann Allergy Clin Immunol. 2015 Mar;47(2):54-7. PubMed PMID: 25781195.

[65] Rodrigo L, Hernández-Lahoz C, Lauret E, Rodriguez-Peláez M, Soucek M, Ciccocioppo R, Kruzliak P. Gluten ataxia is better classified as non-celiac gluten sensitivity than as celiac disease: a comparative clinical study. Immunol Res. 2016 Apr;64(2):558-64. doi: 10.1007/s12026-015-8750-1. PubMed PMID: 26676361.

[66] Makhlouf S, Messelmani M, Zaouali J, Mrissa R. Cognitive impairment in celiac disease and non-celiac gluten sensitivity: review of literature on the main cognitive impairments, the imaging and the effect of gluten free diet. Acta Neurol Belg. 2017 Dec 15. doi: 10.1007/s13760-017-0870-z. [Epub ahead of print] Review. PubMed PMID: 29247390.

[67] Fond G, Boukouaci W, Chevalier G, Regnault A, Eberl G, Hamdani N, Dickerson F, Macgregor A, Boyer L, Dargel A, Oliveira J, Tamouza R, Leboyer M. The "psychomicrobiotic": Targeting microbiota in major psychiatric disorders: A systematic review. Pathol Biol (Paris). 2015 Feb;63(1):35-42. doi: 10.1016/j.patbio.2014.10.003. Epub 2014 Nov 2. Review. PubMed PMID: 25468489.

[68] Justin Hollon, Elaine Leonard Puppa, et al. Effect of Gliadin on Permeability of Intestinal Biopsy Explants from Celiac Disease Patients and Patients with Non-Celiac Gluten Sensitivity. Nutrients. 2015 Mar; 7(3): 1565-1576.

[69] P. Sabelli and P. M. Shewry, "Characterization and Organization of Gene Families at the Gli-1 Loci of Bread and Durum Wheat by Restriction Fragment Analysis," Theoretical and Applied Genetics 83 (1991): 209-16.

[70] Intestinal permeability. (n.d.) Segen's Medical Dictionary. (2011). Retrieved March 6 2018 from //medical-dictionary.thefreedictionary.com/Intestinal+permeability

[71] Maes M, Kubera M, Leunis JC. The gut-brain barrier in major depression: intestinal mucosal dysfunction with an increased translocation of LPS from gram negative enterobacteria (leaky gut) plays a role in the inflammatory pathophysiology of depression. Neuro Endocrinol Lett. 2008 Feb;29(1):117-24. PubMed PMID: 18283240.

[72] "Dermatitis herpetiformis: a cutaneous manifestation of coeliac disease" Ann Med. 2016 Aug 8:1-25

[73] Vassileva S, Drenovska K, Manuelyan K. Autoimmune blistering dermatoses as systemic diseases. Clin Dermatol. 2014 May-Jun;32(3):364-75. doi: 10.1016/j.clindermatol.2013.11.003. Epub 2013 Nov 22. Review. PubMed PMID: 24767184.

[74] Curr Pharm Des. 2014;20(7):1136-8.

[75] "Rapid regression of psoriasis in a coeliac patient after gluten-free diet", Digestion. 2003;68(1):9-12. Epub 2003 Aug 29.

[76] Digestion. 2003;68(1):9-12. Epub 2003 Aug 29.

[77] Pietrzak D, Pietrzak A, Krasowska D, Borzęcki A, Franciszkiewicz-Pietrzak K, Polkowska-Pruszyńska B, Baranowska M, Reich K. Digestive system in psoriasis: an update. Arch Dermatol Res. 2017 Nov;309(9):679-693. doi: 10.1007/s00403-017-1775-7. Epub 2017 Sep 13. Review. PubMed PMID: 28905102; PubMed Central PMCID: PMC5648743.

[78] Kolchak NA, Tetarnikova MK, Theodoropoulou MS, Michalopoulou AP, Theodoropoulos DS. Prevalence of antigliadin IgA antibodies in psoriasis vulgaris and response of seropositive patients to a gluten-free diet. J Multidiscip Healthc. 2017 Dec 27;11:13-19. doi: 10.2147/JMDH.S122256. eCollection 2018. PubMed PMID: 29343966; PubMed Central PMCID: PMC5747961.

[79] Bhatia BK, Millsop JW, Debbaneh M, Koo J, Linos E, Liao W. Diet and psoriasis, part II: celiac disease and role of a gluten-free diet. J Am Acad Dermatol. 2014 Aug;71(2):350-8. doi: 10.1016/j.jaad.2014.03.017. Epub 2014 Apr 26. Review. PubMed PMID: 24780176; PubMed Central PMCID: PMC4104239.

[80] Hindiyeh N, Aurora SK. What the Gut Can Teach Us About Migraine. Curr Pain Headache Rep. 2015 Jul;19(7):33. doi: 10.1007/s11916-015-0501-4. Review. PubMed PMID: 26049770.

[81] Gomes C, Martinho FC, Barbosa DS, Antunes LS, Póvoa HCC, Baltus THL, Morelli NR, Vargas HO, Nunes SOV, Anderson G, Maes M. Increased Root Canal Endotoxin Levels are Associated with Chronic Apical Periodontitis, Increased Oxidative and Nitrosative Stress, Major Depression, Severity of Depression, and a Lowered Quality of Life. Mol Neurobiol. 2018 Apr;55(4):2814-2827. doi: 10.1007/s12035-017-0545-z. Epub 2017 Apr 28. PubMed PMID: 28455694.

[82] Sardu C, Cocco E, Mereu A, Massa R, Cuccu A, Marrosu MG, Contu P. Population based study of 12 autoimmune diseases in Sardinia, Italy: prevalence and comorbidity. PLoS One. 2012;7(3):e32487. doi: 10.1371/journal.pone.0032487. Epub 2012 Mar 2. PubMed PMID: 22396771; PubMed Central PMCID: PMC3292563.

[83] O'Leary C, Walsh CH, Wieneke P, O'Regan P, Buckley B, O'Halloran DJ, Ferriss JB, Quigley EM, Annis P, Shanahan F, Cronin CC. Coeliac disease and autoimmune Addison's disease: a clinical pitfall. QJM. 2002 Feb;95(2):79-82. PubMed PMID: 11861954.

[84] Myhre AG, Aarsetøy H, Undlien DE, Hovdenak N, Aksnes L, Husebye ES. High frequency of coeliac disease among patients with autoimmune adrenocortical failure. Scand J Gastroenterol. 2003 May;38(5):511-5. PubMed PMID: 12795461.

[85] Ch'ng CL, Biswas M, Benton A, Jones MK, Kingham JG. Prospective screening for coeliac disease in patients with Graves' hyperthyroidism using anti-gliadin and tissue transglutaminase antibodies. Clin Endocrinol (Oxf). 2005 Mar;62(3):303-6. Review. PubMed PMID: 15730411.

[86] Page SR, Lloyd CA, Hill PG, Peacock I, Holmes GK. The prevalence of coeliac disease in adult diabetes mellitus. QJM. 1994 Oct;87(10):631-7. PubMed PMID: 7987659.

[87] Ivanova II, Dukova DY, Boikova PG, Grudeva LS, Shalev IB, Kotzev IA. Chronic Hepatitis Due to Gluten Enteropathy - a Case Report. Folia Med (Plovdiv). 2017 Jun 1;59(2):228-231. doi: 10.1515/folmed-2017-0025. PubMed PMID: 28704189.

[88] [Prevalence of gluten-sensitive celiac disease in women with reproductive dysfunction]. Ter Arkh. 2012;84(2):31-6. Russian. PubMed PMID: 22715659.

[89] Ann Neurol 2008;64:332-343

[90] HEPATOLOGY, Vol. 46, No. 5, 2007

[357] Translated by Michael North, National Library of Medicine, 2002.

[358] Green B. Use of the Hippocratic or other professional oaths in UK medical schools in 2017: practice, perception of benefit and principlism. BMC Res Notes. 2017 Dec 29;10(1):777. doi: 10.1186/s13104-017-3114-7. PubMed PMID: 29284529; PubMed Central PMCID: PMC5747024.

[91] R Ciccocioppo, A Di Sabatino, and G R Corazza. "The immune recognition of gluten in coeliac disease" Clin Exp Immunol. 2005 Jun; 140(3): 408-416. doi: 10.1111/j.1365-2249.2005.02783.x

[92] Marsh MN. Gluten, major histocompatibility complex, and the small intestine. A molecular and immunobiologic approach to the spectrum of gluten sensitivity ('celiac sprue').Gastroenterology. 1992 Jan; 102(1):330-54.

[93] Anna Sapone, Julio C Bai, Carolina Ciacci, et al. Spectrum of gluten-related disorders: consensus on new nomenclature and classification. BMC Med. 2012; 10: 13. Published online 2012 Feb 7. doi: 10.1186/1741-7015-10-13. PMCID: PMC3292448

[94] Peña AS, Crusius JB, "Central America in Transition: From Maize to Wheat Challenges and Opportunities", Nutrients. 2015 Aug 26;7(9):7163-71. doi: 10.3390/nu7095330

[95] Evans KE, Hadjivassiliou M, Sanders DS. Recognising coeliac disease in Eastern Europe--the hidden epidemic in our midst? J Gastrointestin Liver Dis. 2011 Jun;20(2):117-8. PubMed PMID: 21725503.

[96] Accomando S, Cataldo F. The global village of celiac disease. Dig Liver Dis. 2004 Jul;36(7):492-8. Review. PubMed PMID: 15285531.

[97] Cataldo F, Montalto G. Celiac disease in the developing countries: a new and challenging public health problem. World J Gastroenterol. 2007 Apr 21;13(15):2153-9. Review. PubMed PMID: 17465493; PubMed Central PMCID: PMC4146836.

[98] Malekzadeh R, Sachdev A, Fahid Ali A. Coeliac disease in developing countries: Middle East, India and North Africa. Best Pract Res Clin Gastroenterol. 2005 Jun;19(3):351-8. Review. PubMed PMID: 15925841.

[99] thisisinsider.com/what-is-gluten-is-it-bad-2018-3

[100] chaunceycrandall.com/food-scams-chauncey-crandall-warns-of-gluten-free-foods

[101] Catassi C, Bearzi I, Holmes GK. Association of celiac disease and intestinal lymphomas and other cancers. Gastroenterology. 2005 Apr;128(4 Suppl 1):S79-86. Review. PubMed PMID: 15825131.

[102] Mangiola F, Ianiro G, Franceschi F, Fagiuoli S, Gasbarrini G, Gasbarrini A. Gut microbiota in autism and mood disorders. World J Gastroenterol. 2016 Jan 7;22(1):361-8. doi: 10.3748/wjg.v22.i1.361. Review. PubMed PMID: 26755882; PubMed Central PMCID: PMC4698498.

[103] statista.com/statistics/307237/otc-sales-in-theus/

[104] World Health Organizatin Fact Sheet: who.int/mediacentre/factsheets/fs369/en/

[105] BMJ Vol.328 21 February 2004 438-9

[106] Dohan F. C., Harper E. H., Clark M. H., Rodrigue R. B., Zigas V. (1984).Is schizophrenia rare if grain is rare?Biol. Psychiatry19, 385-399.

[107] Dohan F. C. (1966a). Wartime changes in hospital admissions for schizophrenia. A comparison of admission for schizophrenia and other psychoses in six countries during World War II. Acta Psychiatr. Scand. 42, 1-23. 10.1111/j.1600-0447.1966.tb01912.x Dohan F. C. (1966b). Wheat "consumption" and hospital admissions for schizophrenia during World War II. A preliminary report. Am. J. Clin. Nutr. 18, 7-10.

[108] Jackson JR, Eaton WW, Cascella NG, Fasano A, Kelly DL. Neurologic and Psychiatric Manifestations of Celiac Disease and Gluten Sensitivity. The Psychiatric quarterly. 2012;83(1):91-102. doi:10.1007/s11126-011-9186-y.

[109] J Int Med. 1997;242:421-423

[110] J Clin Gastroenterol Vol. 42, No. 1, Jan. 2008

[111] Di Lazzaro V, Capone F, Cammarota G, Di Giuda D, Ranieri F. Dramatic improvement of parkinsonian symptoms after gluten-free diet introduction in a patient with silent celiac disease. J Neurol. 2014 Feb;261(2):443-5. doi: 10.1007/s00415-014-7245-7. Epub 2014 Jan 25. PubMed PMID: 24464413.

[112] Hernández-Lahoz C, Rodríguez S, Tuñón A, Saiz A, Santamarta E, Rodrigo L. [Sustained clinical remission in a patient with remittent-recurrent multiple sclerosis and celiac disease gluten-free diet for 6 years]. Neurologia. 2009 Apr;24(3):213-5. Spanish. PubMed PMID: 19418302.

[113] Journal of Attention Disorders, March 2006, 1-5

[114] Yelland GW. Gluten-induced cognitive impairment ("brain fog") in coeliac disease. J Gastroenterol Hepatol. 2017 Mar;32 Suppl 1:90-93. Doi: 10.1111/jgh.13706. Review. PubMed PMID: 28244662.

[115] W. T. Hu et al., "Cognitive Impairment and Celiac Disease," Archives of Neurology 63, no. 10 (October 2006): 1440-46.

[116] Wright DH. The major complications of coeliac disease. Baillieres Clin Gastroenterol. 1995 Jun;9(2):351-69. Review. PubMed PMID: 7549031.

[117] Porcelli, Brunetta et al. "Celiac and Non-Celiac Gluten Sensitivity: A Review on the Association with Schizophrenia and Mood Disorders." Auto-Immunity Highlights 5.2 (2014): 55-61. PMC. Web. 1 Dec. 2017.

[118] Aliment Pharmacol Ther 2002; 16:1333-1339

[119] Lionetti E, Francavilla R, Maiuri L, Ruggieri M, Spina M, Pavone P, Francavilla T, Magistà AM, Pavone L. Headache in pediatric patients with celiac disease and its prevalence as a diagnostic clue. J Pediatr Gastroenterol Nutr. 2009 Aug;49(2):202-7. doi: 10.1097/MPG.0b013e31818f6389. PubMed PMID: 19543115.

[120] Challacombe DN, Wheeler EE. Are the changes of mood in children with coeliac disease due to abnormal serotonin metabolism? Nutr Health. 1987;5(3-4):145-52. Review. PubMed PMID: 3328116.

[121] Choi S, Disilvio B, Fernstrom MH, Fernstrom JD. Meal ingestion, amino acids and brain neurotransmitters: effects of dietary protein source on serotonin and catecholamine synthesis rates. Physiol Behav. 2009 Aug 4;98(1-2):156-62. doi: 10.1016/j.physbeh.2009.05.004. Epub 2009 May 18. PubMed PMID: 19454292.

[122] Fernstrom JD, Langham KA, Marcelino LM, Irvine ZL, Fernstrom MH, Kaye WH. The ingestion of different dietary proteins by humans induces large changes in the plasma tryptophan ratio, a predictor of brain tryptophan uptake and serotonin synthesis. Clin Nutr. 2013 Dec;32(6):1073-6. doi: 10.1016/j.clnu.2012.11.027. Epub 2013 Jan 23. PubMed PMID: 23395255.

[123] Kałuzna-Czaplinska J, Michalska M, Rynkowski J. Determination of tryptophan in urine of autistic and healthy children by gas chromatography/mass spectrometry. Med Sci Monit. 2010 Oct;16(10):CR488-92. PubMed PMID: 20885353.

[124] Kukla U, Łabuzek K, Chronowska J, Krzystanek M, Okopień B. [Mental disorders in digestive system diseases - internist's and psychiatrist's insight]. Pol Merkur Lekarski. 2015 May;38(227):245-9. Polish. PubMed PMID: 26039016.

[125] Aszalós Z. [Neurological and psychiatric aspects of some gastrointestinal diseases]. Orv Hetil. 2008 Nov 2;149(44):2079-86. doi: 10.1556/OH.2008.28480. Review. Hungarian. PubMed PMID: 18952527.

[126] Kowalczyk, Małgorzata Urban. "Psychiatric Complications of Celiac Disease." International Journal of Celiac Disease 3.1 (2015): 25-27.

[127] statcan.gc.ca/pub/82-003-x/2016005/article/14613-eng.htm

[128] Dickerson F, Stallings C, Origoni A, Vaughan C, Khushalani S, Alaedini A, Yolken R. Markers of gluten sensitivity and celiac disease in bipolar disorder. Bipolar Disord. 2011 Feb;13(1):52-8. doi: 10.1111/j.1399-5618.2011.00894.x. PubMed PMID: 21320252.

[129] Dickerson F, Stallings C, Origoni A, Vaughan C, Khushalani S, Leister F, Yang S, Krivogorsky B, Alaedini A, Yolken R. Markers of gluten sensitivity and celiac disease in recent-onset psychosis and multi-episode

schizophrenia. Biol Psychiatry. 2010 Jul 1;68(1):100-4. doi: 10.1016/j.biopsych.2010.03.021. Epub 2010 May 14. PubMed PMID: 20471632.

[130] Samaroo D, Dickerson F, Kasarda DD, Green PH, Briani C, Yolken RH, Alaedini A. Novel immune response to gluten in individuals with schizophrenia. Schizophr Res. 2010 May;118(1-3):248-55. doi: 10.1016/j.schres.2009.08.009. Epub 2009 Sep 11. PubMed PMID: 19748229; PubMed Central PMCID: PMC2856786.

[131] Rowland LM, Demyanovich HK, Wijtenburg SA, Eaton WW, Rodriguez K, Gaston F, Cihakova D, Talor MV, Liu F, McMahon RR, Hong LE, Kelly DL. Antigliadin Antibodies (AGA IgG) Are Related to Neurochemistry in Schizophrenia. Front Psychiatry. 2017 Jun 19;8:104. doi: 10.3389/fpsyt.2017.00104. eCollection 2017. PubMed PMID: 28674504; PubMed Central PMCID: PMC5474459.

[132] Zelnik N, Pacht A, Obeid R, Lerner A. Range of neurologic disorders in patients with celiac disease. Pediatrics. 2004 Jun;113(6):1672-6. PubMed PMID: 15173490

[133] Bingham KS, Rothschild AJ, Mulsant BH, Whyte EM, Meyers BS, Banerjee S, Szanto K, Flint AJ; STOP-PD Study Group. The Association of Baseline Suicidality With Treatment Outcome in Psychotic Depression. J Clin Psychiatry. 2017 Sep/Oct;78(8):1149-1154. doi: 10.4088/JCP.16m10881. PubMed PMID: 28445632.

[134] Rahikainen AL, Majaharju S, Haukka J, Palo JU, Sajantila A. Serotonergic 5HTTLPR/rs25531 s-allele homozygosity associates with violent suicides in male citalopram users. Am J Med Genet B Neuropsychiatr Genet. 2017 Oct;174(7):691-700. doi: 10.1002/ajmg.b.32553. Epub 2017 Jun 13. PubMed PMID: 28608626.

[135] Fazel S, Grann M, Ahlner J, Goodwin G. Suicides by violent means in individuals taking SSRIs and other antidepressants: a postmortem study in Sweden, 1992-2004. J Clin Psychopharmacol. 2007 Oct;27(5):503-6. Erratum in: J Clin Psychopharmacol. 2008 Feb;28(1):123. PubMed PMID: 17873685.

[136] cdc.gov/ncbddd/autism/data.html

[137] Heise CW, Malashock H, Brooks DE. A review of vilazodone exposures with focus on serotonin syndrome effects. Clin Toxicol (Phila). 2017 Nov;55(9):1004-1007. doi: 10.1080/15563650.2017.1332369. Epub 2017 Jun 8. PubMed PMID: 28594246.

[138] Journal of Attention Disorders, March 2006, 1-5

[139] Niederhofer H, Pittschieler K. A preliminary investigation of ADHD symptoms in persons with celiac disease. J Atten Disord. 2006 Nov;10(2):200-4. PubMed PMID: 17085630.

[140] Couture DC, Chung MK, Shinnick P, Curzon J, McClure MJ, LaRiccia PJ. Integrative Medicine Approach to Pediatric Obsessive-Compulsive Disorder and Anxiety: A Case Report. Global Advances in Health and Medicine. 2016;5(1):117-121. doi:10.7453/gahmj.2015.091.

[141] Cade R., Privette M., Fregly M., et al. (2000). Autism and schizophrenia: intestinal disorders. Nutr. Neurosci. 3, 57-72. 10.3109/10284150009163451

[142] Ben Hariz M, Kallel-Sellami M, Kallel L, Lahmer A, Halioui S, Bouraoui S, Laater A, Sliti A, Mahjoub A, Zouari B, Makni S, Maherzi A. Prevalence of celiac disease in Tunisia: mass-screening study in schoolchildren. Eur J Gastroenterol Hepatol. 2007 Aug;19(8):687-94. PubMed PMID: 17625439.

[143] Duerksen DR, Leslie WD. Positive celiac disease serology and reduced bone mineral density in adult women. Can J Gastroenterol. 2010 Feb;24(2):103-7. PubMed PMID: 20151068; PubMed Central PMCID: PMC2852231.

[144] Björck S, Brundin C, Karlsson M, Agardh D. Reduced Bone Mineral Density in Children With Screening-detected Celiac Disease. J Pediatr Gastroenterol Nutr. 2017 Nov;65(5):526-532. doi: 10.1097/MPG.0000000000001568. PubMed PMID: 28319607.

[146] Albulova EA, Drozdov VN, Parfenov AI, Viazhevich IuV, Petrakov AV, Varvanina GG. [Bone mineral density in patients with gluten-sensitivity celiac disease]. Ter Arkh. 2010;82(2):43-8. Russian. PubMed PMID: 20387675.

[147] Dias Costa F, Maia C, Almeida S, Ferreira R. Child with multiple fractures: a rare presentation of a common disease. BMJ Case Rep. 2017 Jan 20;2017. pii: bcr2016218477. doi: 10.1136/bcr-2016-218477. PubMed PMID: 28108441.

[148] Dig Liver Dis 2011 Aug;43(8):616-22

[149] Bender L. Childhood schizophrenia. Psychiatric Quarterly. 1953;27:663-681.

[150] Am J Gastroenterol. 2009 Dec;104(12):3058-67

[151] Sevinç E, Çetin FH, Coşkun BD, "Psychopathology, quality of life, and related factors in children with celiac disease." J Pediatr (Rio J). 2016 Nov 23. pii: S0021-7557(16)30279-0. doi: 10.1016/j.jped.2016.06.012. [Epub ahead of print]

[152] Agnieszka Butwicka MD, PhD, Paul Lichtenstein, PhD, Louise Frisén, MD, PhD, Catarina Almqvist, MD, PhD, Henrik Larsson, PhD, Jonas F. Ludvigsson, MD, PhD. Celiac Disease Is Associated with Childhood Psychiatric Disorders: A Population-Based Study. The Journal of Pediatrics. May 2017 Volume 184, Pages 87-93.e1

[153] Scan J Gastro 2005;40:1407-1412

[154] Al-Hussaini A, Troncone R, Khormi M, AlTuraiki M, Alkhamis W, Alrajhi M, Halal T, Fagih M, Alharbi S, Bashir MS, Chentoufi AA. Mass Screening for Celiac Disease Among School-aged Children: Toward Exploring Celiac Iceberg in Saudi Arabia. J Pediatr Gastroenterol Nutr. 2017 Dec;65(6):646-651. doi: 10.1097/MPG.0000000000001681. PubMed PMID: 28753180.

[155] Du Y, Shan LF, Cao ZZ, Feng JC, Cheng Y. Prevalence of celiac disease in patients with Down syndrome: a meta-analysis. Oncotarget. 2017 Dec 23;9(4):5387-5396. doi: 10.18632/oncotarget.23624. eCollection 2018 Jan 12. PubMed PMID: 29435186; PubMed Central PMCID: PMC5797057.

[156] Bhat AS, Chaturvedi MK, Saini S, Bhatnagar S, Gupta N, Sapra S, Gupta SD, Kabra M. Prevalence of celiac disease in Indian children with Down syndrome and its clinical and laboratory predictors. Indian J Pediatr. 2013 Feb;80(2):114-7. doi: 10.1007/s12098-012-0838-1. Epub 2012 Jul 13. PubMed PMID: 22791400.

[157] SOURCE: India Tribune, Sept 5, 2016, "Celiac disease on rise, state tops list". tribuneindia.com/news/haryana/celiac-disease-on-rise-state-tops-list/290359.html

[158] Cerqueira RM, Rocha CM, Fernandes CD, Correia MR. Celiac disease in Portuguese children and adults with Down syndrome. Eur J Gastroenterol Hepatol. 2010 Jul;22(7):868-71. PubMed PMID: 20545028.

[159] Nisihara RM, Kotze LM, Utiyama SR, Oliveira NP, Fiedler PT, Messias-Reason IT. Celiac disease in children and adolescents with Down syndrome. J Pediatr (Rio J).2005 Sep-Oct;81(5):373-6. PubMed PMID: 16247538.

[160] Lachaux A. Les formes cliniques trompeuses de la maladie cœliaque. Arch Pediatr. 2006 Jun;13(6):572-4.

[161] Solaymani-Dodaran M, West J, Logan RF. Long-term mortality in people with celiac disease diagnosed in childhood compared with adulthood: a population-based cohort study. Am J Gastroenterol. 2007 Apr;102(4):864-70. Epub 2007 Feb 23. PubMed PMID: 17324126.

[162] Hamilton JR, Lynch MJ, Reilly BJ. Active coeliac disease in childhood. Clinical and laboratory findings of forty-two cases. Q J Med. 1969 Apr;38(150):135-58. PubMed PMID: 5781348.

[163] S Igbinedion, J Ansari, et al. World J Gastroenterol. Non-celiac gluten sensitivity: All wheat attack is not celiac. Oct 28, 2017; 23(40): 7201-7210

[164] The American J of Medicine (2006) 119, 355.e9-355.e14

[165] BMJ VOL. 319 24 JULY 1999,236-239

[166] Kieslich,M., Pediatrics Vol.108 No.2, August 2001

[167] Am J Gastroenter, Vol. 98, No 3 2003 626-9

[168] Hemmings W. A. (1978). The entry into the brain of large molecules derived from dietary protein. Proc. R. Soc. Lond. B. Biol. Sci. 200, 175-192. 10.1098/rspb.1978.0014

[169] Hemmings WA. The entry into the brain of large molecules derived from dietary protein. Proc R Soc Lond B Biol Sci. 1978 Feb 23;200(1139):175-92. PubMed PMID: 24851.

[170] Pruimboom L, de Punder K. The opioid effects of gluten exorphins: asymptomatic celiac disease. J Health Popul Nutr. 2015 Nov 24;33:24. doi: 10.1186/s41043-015-0032-y. Review. PubMed PMID: 26825414; PubMed Central PMCID: PMC5025969.

[171] Dr. Daniel Amen, double board-certified psychiatrist, physician, founder of Amen Clinics and BrainMD

[172] Fanciulli G, Dettori A, Demontis MP, Tomasi PA, Anania V, Delitala G. Gluten exorphin B5 stimulates prolactin secretion through opioid receptors located outside the blood-brain barrier. Life Sci. 2005 Feb 25;76(15):1713-9. Epub 2004 Dec 20. PubMed PMID: 15698850.

[173] Fanciulli G, Dettori A, Fenude E, Demontis MP, Alberico E, Delitala G, Anania V. Intravenous administration of the food-derived opioid peptide gluten exorphin B5 stimulates prolactin secretion in rats. Pharmacol Res. 2003 Jan;47(1):53-8. PubMed PMID: 12526862.

[174] Voke J. Pituitary gland: master of the endocrines. Nurs Mirror. 1979 Aug 30;149(9):26-8. PubMed PMID: 257655.

[175] Mitoma H, Manto M, Hampe CS. Time Is Cerebellum. Cerebellum. 2018 Feb 19. doi: 10.1007/s12311-018-0925-6. [Epub ahead of print] PubMed PMID: 29460203.

[176] G. Gobbi et al., "Coeliac Disease, Epilepsy, and Cerebral Calcifications. The Italian Working Group on Coeliac Disease and Epilepsy," Lancet 340, no. 8817 (August 22, 1992): 439-43.

[177] Addolorato G, Mirijello A, D'Angelo C, Leggio L, Ferrulli A, Vonghia L, Cardone S, Leso V, Miceli A, Gasbarrini G. Social phobia in coeliac disease. Scand J Gastroenterol. 2008;43(4):410-5. doi: 10.1080/00365520701768802. PubMed PMID: 18365905.

[178] Brennan KC, Bates EA, Shapiro RE, Zyuzin J, Hallows WC, Huang Y, Lee HY, Jones CR, Fu YH, Charles AC, Ptáček LJ. Casein kinase iδ mutations in familial migraine and advanced sleep phase. Sci Transl Med. 2013 May 1;5(183):183ra56, 1-11. doi: 10.1126/scitranslmed.3005784. PubMed PMID: 23636092; PubMed Central PMCID: PMC4220792.

[179] Severance EG, Gressitt KL, Yang S, Stallings CR, Origoni AE, Vaughan C, Khushalani S, Alaedini A, Dickerson FB, Yolken RH. Seroreactive marker for inflammatory bowel disease and associations with antibodies to dietary proteins in bipolar disorder. Bipolar Disord. 2014 May;16(3):230-40. doi: 10.1111/bdi.12159. Epub 2013 Dec 6. PubMed PMID: 24313887; PubMed Central PMCID: PMC4075657.

[180] Severance EG, Dupont D, Dickerson FB, Stallings CR, Origoni AE, Krivogorsky B, Yang S, Haasnoot W, Yolken RH. Immune activation by casein dietary antigens in bipolar disorder. Bipolar Disord. 2010 Dec;12(8):834-42. doi: 10.1111/j.1399-5618.2010.00879.x. PubMed PMID: 21176030.

[181] Severance EG, Gressitt KL, Halling M, Stallings CR, Origoni AE, Vaughan C, Khushalani S, Alaedini A, Dupont D, Dickerson FB, Yolken RH. Complement C1q formation of immune complexes with milk caseins and wheat glutens in schizophrenia. Neurobiol Dis. 2012 Dec;48(3):447-53. doi: 10.1016/j.nbd.2012.07.005. Epub 2012 Jul 16. PubMed PMID: 22801085; PubMed Central PMCID: PMC3465075.

[182] journals.sagepub.com/doi/abs/10.1177/1362361399003001007

[183] Niebuhr DW, Li Y, Cowan DN, Weber NS, Fisher JA, Ford GM, Yolken R. Association between bovine casein antibody and new onset schizophrenia among US military personnel. Schizophr Res. 2011 May;128(1-3):51-5. doi: 10.1016/j.schres.2011.02.005. Epub 2011 Mar 4. PubMed PMID: 21376538.

[184] Severance EG, Dickerson FB, Halling M, Krivogorsky B, Haile L, Yang S, Stallings CR, Origoni AE, Bossis I, Xiao J, Dupont D, Haasnoot W, Yolken RH. Subunit and whole molecule specificity of the anti-bovine casein immune response in recent onset psychosis and schizophrenia. Schizophr Res. 2010 May;118(1-3):240-7. doi: 10.1016/j.schres.2009.12.030. Epub 2010 Jan 13. PubMed PMID: 20071146.

[185] Tsukahara N, Ezawa I. [Calcium intake and osteoporosis in many countries]. Clin Calcium. 2001 Feb;11(2):173-7. Japanese. PubMed PMID: 15775506.

[186] ARCH INTERN MED/Vol. 165, Feb.28, 2005, 393-399

[187] Benjamin Lebwohl, MD, MS,Columbia University Medical Center

[188] "Villous atrophy in celiac disease linked to hip fracture" Lebwohl B. Su1017: Mucosal Healing and Risk of Fracture in Celiac Disease. Presented at: Digestive Disease Week; May 18-21, Orlando, FL

[189] Tjellström B, Stenhammar L, Sundqvist T, Fälth-Magnusson K, Hollén E, Magnusson KE, Norin E, Midtvedt T, Högberg L. The effects of oats on the function of gut microflora in children with coeliac disease. Aliment Pharmacol Ther. 2014 May;39(10):1156-60. doi: 10.1111/apt.12707. Epub 2014 Mar 24. PubMed PMID: 24661128.

[190] Carlo Catassi, et al., A prospective, double-blind, placebo-controlled trial to establish a safe gluten threshold for patients with celiac disease 1,2,3, American Journal of Clinical Nutrition, Vol. 85, No. 1, 160-166, January 2007

[191] Thies F, Masson LF, Boffetta P, Kris-Etherton P. Oats and bowel disease: a systematic literature review. Br J Nutr. 2014 Oct;112 Suppl 2:S31-43. doi: 10.1017/S0007114514002293. Review. PubMed PMID: 25267242.

[192] I.W. Davidson et al., Clinical and Experimental Immunology 35, No. 1 (Jan 1979): 147-148

[193] J Pediatr Gastroenterol Nutr 1987 May Jun;6(3):346-50

[194] Fernstrom JD, Lytle LD. Corn malnutrition, brain serotonin and behavior. Nutr Rev. 1976 Sep;34(9):257-62. Review. PubMed PMID: 787836.

[195] McDonald's Corporation v Steel & Morris [1997] also known as the McLibel case

[196] R. Gibson, "Zinc Nutrition in Developing Countries," Nutrition Research Reviews 7 (1994): 151-73; L. H. Allen, "The Nutrition CRSP: What Is Marginal Malnutrition and Does It Affect Human Function?" Nutrition Reviews 51 (1993): 255-67.

[197] P. B. Holm, K. N. Kristiansen, and H. B. Pedersen, "Transgenic Approaches in Commonly Consumed Cereals to Improve Iron and Zinc Content and Bioavailability," Journal of Nutrition 132, no. 3 (March 2002): 514S-6S.

[198] V. Lorenzsonn and W. A. Olsen, "In Vivo Responses of Rat Intestinal Epithelium to Intraluminal Dietary Lectins," Gastroenterology 82 (1982): 838-48.

[199] Signorello MG, Leoncini G. The molecular mechanisms involved in lectin-induced human platelet aggregation. Biol Chem. 2017 Nov 27;398(12):1335-1346. Doi: 10.1515/hsz-2017-0115. PubMed PMID: 28779561.

[200] Ohmori T, Yatomi Y, Wu Y, Osada M, Satoh K, Ozaki Y. Wheat germ agglutinin-induced platelet activation via platelet endothelial cell adhesion molecule-1: involvement of rapid phospholipase C gamma 2 activation by Src family kinases. Biochemistry. 2001 Oct 30;40(43):12992-3001. PubMed PMID: 11669637.

[201] Geahlen RL. Getting Syk: Spleen Tyrosine Kinase as a Therapeutic Target. Trends in pharmacological sciences. 2014;35(8):414-422. doi:10.1016/j.tips.2014.05.007.

[202] Laatikainen R, Koskenpato J, Hongisto SM, Loponen J, Poussa T, Huang X, Sontag-Strohm T, Salmenkari H, Korpela R. Pilot Study: Comparison of Sourdough Wheat Bread and Yeast-Fermented Wheat Bread in Individuals with Wheat Sensitivity and Irritable Bowel Syndrome. Nutrients. 2017 Nov 4;9(11). pii: E1215. doi: 10.3390/nu9111215. PubMed PMID: 29113045; PubMed Central PMCID: PMC5707687.

[203] Reig-Otero Y, Mañes J, Manyes L. Amylase-Trypsin Inhibitors in Wheat and Other Cereals as Potential Activators of the Effects of Nonceliac Gluten Sensitivity. J Med Food. 2018 Jan 9. doi: 10.1089/jmf.2017.0018. [Epub ahead of print] PubMed PMID: 29315017.

[204] Schuppan D, Zevallos V. Wheat amylase trypsin inhibitors as nutritional activators of innate immunity. Dig Dis. 2015;33(2):260-3. doi: 10.1159/000371476. Epub 2015 Apr 22. Review. PubMed PMID: 25925932.

[205] Zevallos VF, Raker V, Tenzer S, Jimenez-Calvente C, Ashfaq-Khan M, Rüssel N, Pickert G, Schild H, Steinbrink K, Schuppan D. Nutritional Wheat Amylase-Trypsin Inhibitors Promote Intestinal Inflammation via Activation of Myeloid Cells. Gastroenterology. 2017 Apr;152(5):1100-1113.e12. doi: 10.1053/j.gastro.2016.12.006. Epub 2016 Dec 16. PubMed PMID: 27993525.

[206] Junker Y, Zeissig S, Kim S-J, et al. Wheat amylase trypsin inhibitors drive intestinal inflammation via activation of toll-like receptor 4. The Journal of

Experimental Medicine. 2012;209(13):2395-2408. doi:10.1084/jem.20102660.

[207] Zevallos VF, Raker V, Tenzer S, Jimenez-Calvente C, Ashfaq-Khan M, Rüssel N, Pickert G, Schild H, Steinbrink K, Schuppan D. Nutritional Wheat Amylase-Trypsin Inhibitors Promote Intestinal Inflammation via Activation of Myeloid Cells. Gastroenterology. 2017 Apr;152(5):1100-1113.e12. doi: 10.1053/j.gastro.2016.12.006. Epub 2016 Dec 16. PubMed PMID: 27993525.

[208] Skodje GI, Sarna VK, Minelle IH, Rolfsen KL, Muir JG, Gibson PR, Veierød MB, Henriksen C, Lundin KEA. Fructan, Rather Than Gluten, Induces Symptoms in Patients With Self-Reported Non-Celiac Gluten Sensitivity. Gastroenterology. 2018 Feb;154(3):529-539.e2. doi: 10.1053/j.gastro.2017.10.040. Epub 2017 Nov 2. PubMed PMID: 29102613.

[209] Chumpitazi BP, McMeans AR, Vaughan A, Ali A, Orlando S, Elsaadi A, Shulman RJ. Fructans Exacerbate Symptoms in a Subset of Children With Irritable Bowel Syndrome. Clin Gastroenterol Hepatol. 2018 Feb;16(2):219-225.e1. doi: 10.1016/j.cgh.2017.09.043. Epub 2017 Sep 29. PubMed PMID: 28970147; PubMed Central PMCID: PMC5794652.

[210] Barmeyer C, Schumann M, Meyer T, et al. Long-term response to gluten-free diet as evidence for non-celiac wheat sensitivity in one third of patients with diarrhea-dominant and mixed-type irritable bowel syndrome. International Journal of Colorectal Disease. 2017;32(1):29-39. doi:10.1007/s00384-016-2663-x.

[211] Nijeboer P, Mulder C, Bouma G. [Non-coeliac gluten sensitivity: hype, or new epidemic?]. Ned Tijdschr Geneeskd. 2013;157(21):A6168. Review. Dutch. PubMed PMID: 23693012.

[212] S. S. Mehr et al., "Rice: A Common and Severe Cause of Food Protein-Induced Enterocolitis Syndrome," Archives of Disease in Childhood 94, no. 3 (March 2009): 220-23.

[213] J. R. Lukacs, "Climate, Subsistence, and Health in Prehistoric India," in Ancient Health: Skeletal Indicators of Agricultural and Economic Intensification, ed. M. N. Cohen and G. M. M. Crane-Kramer (Gainesville: University Press of Florida, 2007), 245.

[214] Um MY, Kim S, Jin YH, Yoon M, Yang H, Lee J, Jung J, Urade Y, Huang ZL, Kwon S, Cho S. A novel neurological function of rice bran: a standardized rice bran supplement promotes non-rapid eye movement sleep in mice through histamine H(1) receptors. Mol Nutr Food Res. 2017 Nov;61(11). doi: 10.1002/mnfr.201700316. Epub 2017 Aug 29. PubMed PMID: 28722302.

[215] "Oral manifestations of celiac disease: a clinical guide for dentists" J Mich Dent Assoc. 2011 Oct;93(10):42-6.PMID: 22073722

[216] DiNicolantonio JJ, Mehta V, Onkaramurthy N, O'Keefe JH. Fructose-induced inflammation and increased cortisol: A new mechanism for how sugar induces visceral adiposity. Prog Cardiovasc Dis. 2017 Dec 8. pii: S0033-0620(17)30162-7. doi: 10.1016/j.pcad.2017.12.001. [Epub ahead of print] Review. PubMed PMID: 29225114.

[217] Cigliano L, Spagnuolo MS, Crescenzo R, Cancelliere R, Iannotta L, Mazzoli A, Liverini G, Iossa S. Short-Term Fructose Feeding Induces Inflammation and Oxidative Stress in the Hippocampus of Young and Adult Rats. Mol Neurobiol. 2017 Apr 28. doi: 10.1007/s12035-017-0518-2. [Epub ahead of print] PubMed PMID: 28455700.

[218] Djordjevic A, Bursać B, Veličković N, Vasiljević A, Matić G. The impact of different fructose loads on insulin sensitivity, inflammation, and PSA-

NCAM-mediated plasticity in the hippocampus of fructose-fed male rats. Nutr Neurosci. 2015 Feb;18(2):66-75. doi: 10.1179/1476830513Y.0000000098. Epub 2013 Nov 25. PubMed PMID: 24257416.

[219] Rippe JM, Angelopoulos TJ. Relationship between Added Sugars Consumption and Chronic Disease Risk Factors: Current Understanding. Nutrients. 2016 Nov 4;8(11). pii: E697. Review. PubMed PMID: 27827899; PubMed Central PMCID: PMC5133084.

[220] Hsu TM, Konanur VR, Taing L, Usui R, Kayser BD, Goran MI, Kanoski SE. Effects of sucrose and high fructose corn syrup consumption on spatial memory function and hippocampal neuroinflammation in adolescent rats. Hippocampus. 2015 Feb;25(2):227-39. doi: 10.1002/hipo.22368. Epub 2014 Oct 3. PubMed PMID: 25242636.

[221] Belloir C, Neiers F, Briand L. Sweeteners and sweetness enhancers. Curr Opin Clin Nutr Metab Care. 2017 Jul;20(4):279-285. doi: 10.1097/MCO.0000000000000377. Review. PubMed PMID: 28399012.

[222] Sharma A, Amarnath S, Thulasimani M, Ramaswamy S. Artificial sweeteners as a sugar substitute: Are they really safe? Indian J Pharmacol. 2016 May-Jun;48(3):237-40. doi: 10.4103/0253-7613.182888. PubMed PMID: 27298490; PubMed Central PMCID: PMC4899993.

[223] Laffitte A, Neiers F, Briand L. Functional roles of the sweet taste receptor in oral and extraoral tissues. Curr Opin Clin Nutr Metab Care. 2014 Jul;17(4):379-85. doi: 10.1097/MCO.0000000000000058. Review. PubMed PMID: 24763065; PubMed Central PMCID: PMC4059820.

[224] Neiers F, Canivenc-Lavier MC, Briand L. What Does Diabetes "Taste" Like? Curr Diab Rep. 2016 Jun;16(6):49. doi: 10.1007/s11892-016-0746-2. Review. PubMed PMID: 27085864.

[225] Hooshmand S, Holloway B, Nemoseck T, Cole S, Petrisko Y, Hong MY, Kern M. Effects of agave nectar versus sucrose on weight gain, adiposity, blood glucose, insulin, and lipid responses in mice. J Med Food. 2014 Sep;17(9):1017-21. doi: 10.1089/jmf.2013.0162. Epub 2014 Jul 10. PubMed PMID: 25011004.

[226] Santos-Zea L, Rosas-Pérez AM, Leal-Díaz AM, Gutiérrez-Uribe JA. Variability in Saponin Content, Cancer Antiproliferative Activity and Physicochemical Properties of Concentrated Agave Sap. J Food Sci. 2016 Aug;81(8):H2069-75. doi: 10.1111/1750-3841.13376. Epub 2016 Jul 4. PubMed PMID: 27376349.

[227] Martineau D, Lemberger K, Dallaire A, et al. Cancer in wildlife, a case study: beluga from the St. Lawrence estuary, Québec, Canada. Environmental Health Perspectives. 2002;110(3):285-292.

[228] Jennings WC, Chern EC, O'Donohue D, Kellogg MG, Boehm AB. Frequent detection of a human fecal indicator in the urban ocean: environmental drivers and covariation with enterococci. Environ Sci Process Impacts. 2018 Feb 6. doi: 10.1039/c7em00594f. [Epub ahead of print] PubMed PMID: 29404550.

[229] Brown TM, Macdonald RW, Muir DCG, Letcher RJ. The distribution and trends of persistent organic pollutants and mercury in marine mammals from Canada's Eastern Arctic. Sci Total Environ. 2018 Mar 15;618:500-517. doi: 10.1016/j.scitotenv.2017.11.052. Epub 2017 Nov 13. Review. PubMed PMID: 29145101.

[230] "The Nobel Prize in Physiology or Medicine 1948". Nobelprize.org. Nobel Media AB 2014.

231 Landsberg JH, Hall S, Johannessen JN, et al. Saxitoxin Puffer Fish Poisoning in the United States, with the First Report of Pyrodinium bahamense as the Putative Toxin Source. Environmental Health Perspectives. 2006;114(10):1502-1507. doi:10.1289/ehp.8998.

232 Grattan LM, Holobaugh S, Morris JG. Harmful Algal Blooms and Public Health. Harmful algae. 2016;57(B):2-8. doi:10.1016/j.hal.2016.05.003.

233 Jones ER, Martyniuk CJ, Morris JM, Krasnec MO, Griffitt RJ. Exposure to Deepwater Horizon oil and Corexit 9500 at low concentrations induces transcriptional changes and alters immune transcriptional pathways in sheepshead minnows. Comp Biochem Physiol Part D Genomics Proteomics. 2017 Sep;23:8-16. doi: 10.1016/j.cbd.2017.05.001. Epub 2017 May 26. PubMed PMID: 28578262.

234 Vignier J, Soudant P, Chu FL, Morris JM, Carney MW, Lay CR, Krasnec MO, Robert R, Volety AK. Lethal and sub-lethal effects of Deepwater Horizon slick oil and dispersant on oyster (Crassostrea virginica) larvae. Mar Environ Res. 2016 Sep;120:20-31. doi: 10.1016/j.marenvres.2016.07.006. Epub 2016 Jul 6. PubMed PMID: 27423003.

235 Collin A. Eagles-Smith, Ellen K. Silbergeld, et al. Modulators of mercury risk to wildlife and humans in the context of rapid global change. Ambio 2018, 47:170-197 DOI 10.1007/s13280-017-1011-x

236 Pigatto PD, Costa A, Guzzi G. Are mercury and Alzheimer's disease linked? Sci Total Environ. 2018 Feb 1;613-614:1579-1580. Doi: 10.1016/j.scitotenv.2017.09.036. Epub 2017 Sep 8. PubMed PMID: 28889904.

237 Tsuda T, Yorifuji T, Takao S, Miyai M, Babazono A. Minamata disease: catastrophic poisoning due to a failed public health response. J Public Health Policy. 2009 Apr;30(1):54-67. doi: 10.1057/jphp.2008.30. PubMed PMID: 19367301.

238 Jovanović B. Ingestion of microplastics by fish and its potential consequences from a physical perspective. Integr Environ Assess Manag. 2017 May;13(3):510-515. doi: 10.1002/ieam.1913. PubMed PMID: 28440941.

239 Jabeen K, Su L, Li J, Yang D, Tong C, Mu J, Shi H. Microplastics and mesoplastics in fish from coastal and fresh waters of China. Environ Pollut. 2017 Feb;221:141-149. doi: 10.1016/j.envpol.2016.11.055. Epub 2016 Dec 7. PubMed PMID: 27939629.

240 Eerkes-Medrano D, Thompson RC, Aldridge DC. Microplastics in freshwater systems: a review of the emerging threats, identification of knowledge gaps and prioritisation of research needs. Water Res. 2015 May 15;75:63-82. doi: 10.1016/j.watres.2015.02.012. Epub 2015 Feb 17. Review. PubMed PMID: 25746963.

241 Sruthy S, Ramasamy EV. Microplastic pollution in Vembanad Lake, Kerala, India: The first report of microplastics in lake and estuarine sediments in India. Environ Pollut. 2017 Mar;222:315-322. doi: 10.1016/j.envpol.2016.12.038. Epub 2016 Dec 29. PubMed PMID: 28041839.

242 Nor NH, Obbard JP. Microplastics in Singapore's coastal mangrove ecosystems. Mar Pollut Bull. 2014 Feb 15;79(1-2):278-83. doi: 10.1016/j.marpolbul.2013.11.025. Epub 2013 Dec 21. PubMed PMID: 24365455.

243 Ballent A, Corcoran PL, Madden O, Helm PA, Longstaffe FJ. Sources and sinks of microplastics in Canadian Lake Ontario nearshore, tributary and beach sediments. Mar Pollut Bull. 2016 Sep 15;110(1):383-395. doi: 10.1016/j.marpolbul.2016.06.037. Epub 2016 Jun 21. PubMed PMID: 27342902.

244 Frias JP, Gago J, Otero V, Sobral P. Microplastics in coastal sediments from Southern Portuguese shelf waters. Mar Environ Res. 2016 Mar;114:24-30. doi: 10.1016/j.marenvres.2015.12.006. Epub 2015 Dec 21. PubMed PMID: 26748246.

245 Castillo AB, Al-Maslamani I, Obbard JP. Prevalence of microplastics in the marine waters of Qatar. Mar Pollut Bull. 2016 Oct 15;111(1-2):260-267. doi: 10.1016/j.marpolbul.2016.06.108. Epub 2016 Jul 4. PubMed PMID: 27389452.

246 Claessens M, De Meester S, Van Landuyt L, De Clerck K, Janssen CR. Occurrence and distribution of microplastics in marine sediments along the Belgian coast. Mar Pollut Bull. 2011 Oct;62(10):2199-204. doi: 10.1016/j.marpolbul.2011.06.030. Epub 2011 Jul 28. PubMed PMID: 21802098.

248 Leslie HA, Brandsma SH, van Velzen MJ, Vethaak AD. Microplastics en route: Field measurements in the Dutch river delta and Amsterdam canals, wastewater treatment plants, North Sea sediments and biota. Environ Int. 2017 Apr;101:133-142. doi: 10.1016/j.envint.2017.01.018. Epub 2017 Jan 28. PubMed PMID: 28143645.

249 Vaughan R, Turner SD, Rose NL. Microplastics in the sediments of a UK urban lake. Environ Pollut. 2017 Oct;229:10-18. doi: 10.1016/j.envpol.2017.05.057. Epub 2017 May 30. PubMed PMID: 28575711.

250 Jansen MD, Bang Jensen B, McLoughlin MF, Rodger HD, Taksdal T, Sindre H, Graham DA, Lillehaug A. The epidemiology of pancreas disease in salmonid aquaculture: a summary of the current state of knowledge. J Fish Dis. 2017 Jan;40(1):141-155. doi: 10.1111/jfd.12478. Epub 2016 May 2. Review. PubMed PMID: 27136332.

251 Madhun AS, Isachsen CH, Omdal LM, Bårdsgjære Einen AC, Bjørn PA, Nilsen R, Karlsbakk E. Occurrence of salmonid alphavirus (SAV) and piscine orthoreovirus (PRV) infections in wild sea trout Salmo trutta in Norway. Dis Aquat Organ. 2016 Jul 7;120(2):109-13. doi: 10.3354/dao03009. PubMed PMID: 27409234.

252 Madhun AS, Isachsen CH, Omdal LM, Einen ACB, Maehle S, Wennevik V, Niemelä E, Svåsand T, Karlsbakk E. Prevalence of piscine orthoreovirus and salmonid alphavirus in sea-caught returning adult Atlantic salmon (Salmo salar L.) in northern Norway. J Fish Dis. 2018 Jan 31. doi: 10.1111/jfd.12785. [Epub ahead of print] PubMed PMID: 29388217.

253 worldgastroenterology.org/wgo-foundation/your-digestive-health

254 Gupta R, Reddy DN, Makharia GK, et al. Indian task force for celiac disease: Current status. World Journal of Gastroenterology: WJG. 2009;15(48):6028-6033. doi:10.3748/wjg.15.6028.

255 scientificamerican.com/article/newborn-babies-chemicals-exposure-bpa/

256 Kershen DL. Health and food safety: the benefits of Bt-corn. Food Drug Law J. 2006;61(2):197-235. PubMed PMID: 16903029.

257 Alzheimer's Association. 2016 Alzheimer's disease facts and figures. Alzheimers Dement. 2016 Apr;12(4):459-509. PubMed PMID: 27570871.

258 S. Boyd Eaton, M.D., Melvin Konner, Ph.D, Paleolithic Nutrition – A Consideration of Its Nature and Current Implications. N Engl J Med 1985; 312:283-289 DOI: 10.1056/NEJM198501313120505

259 Mackarness R., Stone age diet for functional disorders. Med World. 1959 Jul;91:14-9. PMID: 14419471

[260] Davis DL. Paleolithic diet, evolution, and carcinogens. Science. 1987 Dec 18;238(4834):1633-4. PubMed PMID: 3120316.

[261] P. Carrera-Bastos et al., "The Western Diet and Lifestyle and Diseases of Civilization," Research Reports in Clinical Cardiology 2 (2011): 15-35.

[262] Gikas A, Lambadiari V, Sotiropoulos A, Panagiotakos D, Pappas S. Prevalence of Major Cardiovascular Risk Factors and Coronary Heart Disease in a Sample of Greek Adults: The Saronikos Study. The Open Cardiovascular Medicine Journal. 2016;10:69-80. doi:10.2174/1874192401610010069.

[263] Alan M. Friedlander, Enric Ballesteros, et al. Marine biodiversity at the end of the world: Cape Horn and Diego Ramírez islands. PLoS One. 2018; 13(1): e0189930. Published online 2018 Jan 24. doi: 10.1371/journal.pone.0189930

[264] Jung UJ, Kim SR. Beneficial Effects of Flavonoids Against Parkinson's Disease. J Med Food. 2018 Feb 7. doi: 10.1089/jmf.2017.4078. [Epub ahead of print] PubMed PMID: 29412767.

[265] Ma Y, Ma B, Shang Y, Yin Q, Hong Y, Xu S, Shen C, Hou X, Liu X. Flavonoid-rich ethanol extract from the leaves of Diospyros kaki attenuates cognitive deficits, amyloid-beta production, oxidative stress, and neuroinflammation in APP/PS1 transgenic mice. Brain Res. 2018 Jan 1;1678:85-93. Doi: 10.1016/j.brainres.2017.10.001. Epub 2017 Oct 14. PubMed PMID: 29038004.

[266] Spencer JP. The impact of fruit flavonoids on memory and cognition. Br J Nutr. 2010 Oct;104 Suppl 3:S40-7. doi: 10.1017/S0007114510003934. Review. PubMed PMID: 20955649.

[267] Zhang C, Zhou Q, Wu XN, Huang YS, Zhou J, Lai Z, Wu Y, Luo HB. Discovery of novel PDE9A inhibitors with antioxidant activities for treatment of Alzheimer's disease. J Enzyme Inhib Med Chem. 2018 Dec;33(1):260-270. doi: 10.1080/14756366.2017.1412315. PubMed PMID: 29271265.

[268] Rajfer J. Pomegranate Juice: Is It the New, All-Natural Phosphodiesterase Type 5 Inhibitor? Reviews in Urology. 2008;10(2):168-169.

[269] Parasram K. Phytochemical treatments target kynurenine pathway induced oxidative stress. Redox Rep. 2018 Dec;23(1):25-28. doi: 10.1080/13510002.2017.1343223. Epub 2017 Jun 26. PubMed PMID: 28651456.

[270] Granholm AC, Bimonte-Nelson HA, Moore AB, Nelson ME, Freeman LR, Sambamurti K. Effects of a saturated fat and high cholesterol diet on memory and hippocampal morphology in the middle-aged rat. J Alzheimers Dis. 2008 Jun;14(2):133-45. PubMed PMID: 18560126; PubMed Central PMCID: PMC2670571.

[271] Ginter E, Simko V. New data on harmful effects of trans-fatty acids. Bratisl Lek Listy. 2016;117(5):251-3. Review. PubMed PMID: 27215959.

[272] Institute of Medicine (US) Committee on Use of Dietary Reference Intakes in Nutrition Labeling. Dietary Reference Intakes: Guiding Principles for Nutrition Labeling and Fortification. Washington (DC): National Academies Press (US); 2003. 3, Overview of Food Fortification in the United States and Canada.

[273] Park YK, Sempos CT, Barton CN, Vanderveen JE, Yetley EA. Effectiveness of food fortification in the United States: the case of pellagra. Am J Public

Health. 2000 May;90(5):727-38. PubMed PMID: 10800421; PubMed Central PMCID: PMC1446222.

274 Matapandeu G, Dunn SH, Pagels P. An Outbreak of Pellagra in the Kasese Catchment Area, Dowa, Malawi. Am J Trop Med Hyg. 2017 May;96(5):1244-1247. doi: 10.4269/ajtmh.16-0423. Epub 2017 May 13. PubMed PMID: 28219990; PubMed Central PMCID: PMC5417224.

275 CORN treatment and pellagra. Nutr Rev. 1952 Apr;10(4):105-7. PubMed PMID: 14941528.

276 PELLAGRA and the cooking of corn. Nutr Rev. 1957 Feb;15(2):53-5. PubMed PMID: 13400413.

277 LA CAVA AF. [Two communications on Indian corn and pellagra by Carlo Buccio at the Accademia bresciana in 1804 and 1805]. Rass Clin Ter. 1951 Oct-Dec;50(4):Suppl 175-84. Undetermined Language. PubMed PMID: 14920721.

278 Crider KS, Bailey LB, Berry RJ. Folic Acid Food Fortification—Its History, Effect, Concerns, and Future Directions. Nutrients. 2011;3(3):370-384. doi:10.3390/nu3030370.

279 Morris M.S., Jacques P.F., Rosenberg I.H., Selhub J. Circulating unmetabolized folic acid and 5-methyltetrahydrofolate in relation to anemia, macrocytosis, and cognitive test performance in American seniors. Am. J. Clin. Nutr. 2010;91:1733-1744. doi: 10.3945/ajcn.2009.28671.

280 Campbell RK. The unnecessary epidemic of folic acid-preventable spina bifida and anencephaly. Pediatrics. 2001 Oct;108(4):1048-50. PubMed PMID: 11589212.

281 Ren RJ, Wang LL, Fang R, Liu LH, Wang Y, Tang HD, Deng YL, Xu W, Wang G, Chen SD. The MTHFD1L gene rs11754661 marker is associated with susceptibility to Alzheimer's disease in the Chinese Han population. J Neurol Sci. 2011 Sep 15;308(1-2):32-4. doi: 10.1016/j.jns.2011.06.036. Epub 2011 Jul 8. PubMed PMID: 21741665.

282 Bell KN, Oakley GP Jr. Update on prevention of folic acid-preventable spina bifida and anencephaly. Birth Defects Res A Clin Mol Teratol. 2009 Jan;85(1):102-7. doi: 10.1002/bdra.20504. PubMed PMID: 19067404.

283 Centers for Disease Control and Prevention (CDC). Spina bifida and anencephaly before and after folic acid mandate--United States, 1995-1996 and 1999-2000. MMWR Morb Mortal Wkly Rep. 2004 May 7;53(17):362-5. PubMed PMID: 15129193.

284 De Steur H, Mehta S, Gellynck X, Finkelstein JL. GM biofortified crops: potential effects on targeting the micronutrient intake gap in human populations. Curr Opin Biotechnol. 2017 Apr;44:181-188. doi: 10.1016/j.copbio.2017.02.003. Epub 2017 Mar 11. Review. PubMed PMID: 28288329.

285 Petra AI, Panagiotidou S, Hatziagelaki E, Stewart JM, Conti P, Theoharides TC. Gut-Microbiota-Brain Axis and Its Effect on Neuropsychiatric Disorders With Suspected Immune Dysregulation. Clin Ther. 2015 May 1;37(5):984-95. doi: 10.1016/j.clinthera.2015.04.002. Review. PubMed PMID: 26046241; PubMed Central PMCID: PMC4458706.

286 Severance EG, Alaedini A, Yang S, Halling M, Gressitt KL, Stallings CR, Origoni AE, Vaughan C, Khushalani S, Leweke FM, Dickerson FB, Yolken RH. Gastrointestinal inflammation and associated immune activation in schizophrenia. Schizophr Res. 2012 Jun;138(1):48-53. doi:

10.1016/j.schres.2012.02.025. Epub 2012 Mar 24. PubMed PMID: 22446142; Pubmed Central PMCID: PMC4244845.

[287] Kanchanatawan B, Tangwongchai S, Sughondhabhirom A, Suppapitiporn S, Hemrunrojn S, Carvalho AF, Maes M. Add-on Treatment with Curcumin Has Antidepressive Effects in Thai Patients with Major Depression: Results of a Randomized Double-Blind Placebo-Controlled Study. Neurotox Res. 2018 Apr;33(3):621-633. doi: 10.1007/s12640-017-9860-4. Epub 2018 Jan 11. PubMed PMID: 29327213.

[288] Lopresti AL. Curcumin for neuropsychiatric disorders: a review of in vitro, animal and human studies. J Psychopharmacol. 2017 Mar;31(3):287-302. doi: 10.1177/0269881116686883. Epub 2017 Jan 30. Review. PubMed PMID: 28135888.

[289] Kocaadam B, Şanlier N. Curcumin, an active component of turmeric (Curcuma longa), and its effects on health. Crit Rev Food Sci Nutr. 2017 Sep 2;57(13):2889-2895. doi: 10.1080/10408398.2015.1077195. Review. PubMed PMID: 26528921.

[290] Venigalla M, Gyengesi E, Münch G. Curcumin and Apigenin - novel and promising therapeutics against chronic neuroinflammation in Alzheimer's disease. Neural Regen Res. 2015 Aug;10(8):1181-5. doi: 10.4103/1673-5374.162686. Review. Erratum in: Neural Regen Res. 2015 Dec;10(12):2017. PubMed PMID: 26487830; PubMed Central PMCID: PMC4590215.

[291] Whyte AR, Williams CM. Effects of a single dose of a flavonoid-rich blueberry drink on memory in 8 to 10 y old children. Nutrition. 2015 Mar;31(3):531-4. doi: 10.1016/j.nut.2014.09.013. Epub 2014 Oct 18. PubMed PMID: 25701345.

[292] Whyte AR, Schafer G, Williams CM. Cognitive effects following acute wild blueberry supplementation in 7- to 10-year-old children. Eur J Nutr. 2016 Sep;55(6):2151-62. doi: 10.1007/s00394-015-1029-4. Epub 2015 Oct 5. PubMed PMID: 26437830.

[293] Khalid S, Barfoot KL, May G, Lamport DJ, Reynolds SA, Williams CM. Effects of Acute Blueberry Flavonoids on Mood in Children and Young Adults. Nutrients. 2017 Feb 20;9(2). pii: E158. doi: 10.3390/nu9020158. PubMed PMID: 28230732; PubMed Central PMCID: PMC5331589.

[294] Wakimoto R, Ono M, Takeshima M, Higuchi T, Nakano S. Differential Anticancer Activity of Pterostilbene Against Three Subtypes of Human Breast Cancer Cells. Anticancer Res. 2017 Nov;37(11):6153-6159. PubMed PMID: 29061796.

[295] Kosuru R, Rai U, Prakash S, Singh A, Singh S. Promising therapeutic potential of pterostilbene and its mechanistic insight based on preclinical evidence. Eur J Pharmacol. 2016 Oct 15;789:229-243. doi: 10.1016/j.ejphar.2016.07.046. Epub 2016 Jul 27. Review. PubMed PMID: 27475678.

[296] MITCHELL, H. H.; HAMILTON, T. S.; STEGGERDA, F. R.; BEAN, H. W.. Author Affiliation : Div. Animal Nntrit., Univ. Illinois, Urbana. Journal article : Journal of Biological Chemistry 1945 Vol.168 pp.625-637

[297] Benton D, Young HA. Do small differences in hydration status affect mood and mental performance? Nutr Rev. 2015 Sep;73 Suppl 2:83-96. doi: 10.1093/nutrit/nuv045. Review. PubMed PMID: 26290294.

[298] Pross N. Effects of Dehydration on Brain Functioning: A Life-Span Perspective. Ann Nutr Metab. 2017;70 Suppl 1:30-36. doi: 10.1159/000463060. Epub 2017 Jun 15. PubMed PMID: 28614811.

[299] Kleiner SM. Water: an essential but overlooked nutrient. J Am Diet Assoc. 1999 Feb;99(2):200-6. Review. Erratum in: J Am Diet Assoc 1999 Apr;99(4):411. PubMed PMID: 9972188.

[300] Lakhan SE, Vieira KF. Nutritional therapies for mental disorders. Nutr J. 2008 Jan 21;7:2. doi: 10.1186/1475-2891-7-2. Review. PubMed PMID: 18208598; PubMed Central PMCID: PMC2248201.

[301] de Wilde MC, Vellas B, Girault E, Yavuz AC, Sijben JW. Lower brain and blood nutrient status in Alzheimer's disease: Results from meta-analyses. Alzheimers Dement (N Y). 2017 Jun 24;3(3):416-431. doi: 10.1016/j.trci.2017.06.002. eCollection 2017 Sep. Review. PubMed PMID: 29067348; PubMed Central PMCID: PMC5651428.

[302] Cacciatore I, Marinelli L, Fornasari E, Cerasa LS, Eusepi P, Türkez H, Pomilio C, Reale M, D'Angelo C, Costantini E, Di Stefano A. Novel NSAID-Derived Drugs for the Potential Treatment of Alzheimer's Disease. Int J Mol Sci. 2016 Jun 30;17(7). pii: E1035. doi: 10.3390/ijms17071035. PubMed PMID: 27376271; PubMed Central PMCID: PMC4964411.

[303] O. Jokinen et al., "Lectin Binding to the Porcine and Human Ileal Receptor of Intrinsic Factor-Cobalamin," Glycoconjugate Journal 6, no. 4 (1989): 525-38.

[304] Rosenberg IH, Miller JW. Nutritional factors in physical and cognitive functions of elderly people. Am J Clin Nutr. 1992 Jun;55(6 Suppl):1237S-1243S. Review. PubMed PMID: 1590263.

[305] Jay AM, Conway RL, Feldman GL, Nahhas F, Spencer L, Wolf B. Outcomes of individuals with profound and partial biotinidase deficiency ascertained by newborn screening in Michigan over 25 years. Genet Med. 2015 Mar;17(3):205-9. doi: 10.1038/gim.2014.104. Epub 2014 Aug 21. PubMed PMID: 25144890.

[306] Ajith TA, Padmajanair G. Mitochondrial Pharmaceutics: A New Therapeutic Strategy to Ameliorate Oxidative Stress in Alzheimer's Disease. Curr Aging Sci. 2015;8(3):235-40. Review. PubMed PMID: 25986626.

[307] Riedel WJ, Jorissen BL. Nutrients, age and cognitive function. Curr Opin Clin Nutr Metab Care. 1998 Nov;1(6):579-85. Review. PubMed PMID: 10565413.

[308] Harnett NG, Wood KH, Ference EW 3rd, Reid MA, Lahti AC, Knight AJ, Knight DC. Glutamate/glutamine concentrations in the dorsal anterior cingulate vary with Post-Traumatic Stress Disorder symptoms. J Psychiatr Res. 2017 Aug;91:169-176. doi: 10.1016/j.jpsychires.2017.04.010. Epub 2017 Apr 28. PubMed PMID: 28478230.

[309] Rae CD, Williams SR. Glutathione in the human brain: Review of its roles and measurement by magnetic resonance spectroscopy. Anal Biochem. 2017 Jul 15;529:127-143. doi: 10.1016/j.ab.2016.12.022. Epub 2016 Dec 26. Review. PubMed PMID: 28034792.

[310] Reeves JL, Otahal P, Magnussen CG, Dwyer T, Kangas AJ, Soininen P, Ala-Korpela M, Venn AJ, Smith KJ. DHA mediates the protective effect of fish consumption on new episodes of depression among women. Br J Nutr. 2017 Nov;118(9):743-749. doi: 10.1017/S0007114517002768. PubMed PMID: 29185935.

[311] Tesei A, Crippa A, Ceccarelli SB, Mauri M, Molteni M, Agostoni C, Nobile M.The potential relevance of docosahexaenoic acid and eicosapentaenoic acid to the etiopathogenesis of childhood neuropsychiatric disorders. Eur

Child Adolesc Psychiatry. 2017 Sep;26(9):1011-1030. doi: 10.1007/s00787-016-0932-4. Epub 2016 Dec 17. Review. PubMed PMID: 27988864.

[312] Conlon MA, Bird AR. The Impact of Diet and Lifestyle on Gut Microbiota and Human Health. Nutrients. 2015;7(1):17-44. doi:10.3390/nu7010017.

[313] Harper A, Naghibi MM, Garcha D. The Role of Bacteria, Probiotics and Diet in Irritable Bowel Syndrome. Foods. 2018 Jan 26;7(2). pii: E13. doi: 10.3390/foods7020013. Review. PubMed PMID: 29373532; PubMed Central PMCID: PMC5848117.

[314] Yang Y, Tian J, Yang B. Targeting gut microbiome: A novel and potential therapy for autism. Life Sci. 2018 Feb 1;194:111-119. doi: 10.1016/j.lfs.2017.12.027. Epub 2017 Dec 23. Review. PubMed PMID: 29277311.

[315] Tompkins TA, Mainville I, Arcand Y. The impact of meals on a probiotic during transit through a model of the human upper gastrointestinal tract. Benef Microbes. 2011 Dec 1;2(4):295-303. doi: 10.3920/BM2011.0022. PubMed PMID: 22146689.

[316] Postgrad Med J 2002;78:31-33

[317] Sofi F, Valecchi D, Bacci D, Abbate R, Gensini GF, Casini A, Macchi C. Physical activity and risk of cognitive decline: a meta-analysis of prospective studies. J Intern Med. 2011 Jan;269(1):107-17. doi: 10.1111/j.1365-2796.2010.02281.x. Epub 2010 Sep 10. Review. PubMed PMID: 20831630.

[318] Laurin D, Verreault R, Lindsay J, MacPherson K, Rockwood K. Physical activity and risk of cognitive impairment and dementia in elderly persons. Arch Neurol. 2001 Mar;58(3):498-504. PubMed PMID: 11255456.

[319] Yaffe K, Barnes D, Nevitt M, Lui LY, Covinsky K. A prospective study of physical activity and cognitive decline in elderly women: women who walk. Arch Intern Med. 2001 Jul 23;161(14):1703-8. PubMed PMID: 11485502.

[320] Russell-Williams J, Jaroudi W, Perich T, Hoscheidt S, El Haj M, Moustafa AA.Mindfulness and meditation: treating cognitive impairment and reducing stress in dementia. Rev Neurosci. 2018 Feb 21. pii: /j/revneuro.ahead-of-print/revneuro-2017-0066/revneuro-2017-0066.xml. doi:10.1515/revneuro-2017-0066. [Epub ahead of print] PubMed PMID: 29466242.

[321] Wells RE, Yeh GY, Kerr CE, Wolkin J, Davis RB, Tan Y, Spaeth R, Wall RB, Walsh J, Kaptchuk TJ, Press D, Phillips RS, Kong J. Meditation's impact on default mode network and hippocampus in mild cognitive impairment: a pilot study. Neurosci Lett. 2013 Nov 27;556:15-9. doi: 10.1016/j.neulet.2013.10.001. Epub 2013 Oct 10. PubMed PMID: 24120430; PubMed Central PMCID: PMC4022038.

[322] Conklin QA, King BG, Zanesco AP, Lin J, Hamidi AB, Pokorny JJ, Jesús Álvarez-López M, Cosín-Tomás M, Huang C, Kaliman P, Epel ES, Saron CD. Insight
Meditation and Telomere Biology: The Effects of Intensive Retreat and the Moderating Role of Personality. Brain Behav Immun. 2018 Mar 5. pii: S0889-1591(18)30047-3. doi: 10.1016/j.bbi.2018.03.003. [Epub ahead of print] PubMed PMID: 29518528.

[323] Househam AM, Peterson CT, Mills PJ, Chopra D. The Effects of Stress and Meditation on the Immune System, Human Microbiota, and Epigenetics. Adv Mind Body Med. 2017 Fall;31(4):10-25. PubMed PMID: 29306937.

[324] American Autoimmune Related Diseases Association, 22100 Gratiot Avenue, Eastpointe, MI 48021-2227 www.aarda.org

[325] Troncone R, Auricchio R, Granata V., Issues related to gluten-free diet in coeliac disease., Department of Pediatrics and European Laboratory for the Investigation of Food-Induced Diseases, University Federico II, Naples, Italy., Curr Opin Clin Nutr Metab Care. 2008 May;11(3):329-33.

[326] Akobeng AK, Thomas AG., Systematic review: tolerable amount of gluten for people with coeliac disease., Department of Paediatric Gastroenterology, Booth Hall Children's Hospital, Central Manchester and Manchester Children's University Hospitals, Manchester, UK., Aliment Pharmacol Ther. 2008 Jun 1;27(11):1044-52. Epub 2008 Feb 29.

[327] Carlo Catassi, et al., A prospective, double-blind, placebo-controlled trial to establish a safe gluten threshold for patients with celiac disease 1,2,3, American Journal of Clinical Nutrition, Vol. 85, No. 1, 160-166, January 2007

[328] C. Zioudrou, R. A. Streaty, and W. A. Klee, "Opioid Peptides Derived from Food Proteins. The Exorphins," Journal of Biological Chemistry 254, no. 7 (April 10, 1979): 2446–49.

[329] Sokolov O, Kost N, Andreeva O, Korneeva E, Meshavkin V, Tarakanova Y, Dadayan A, Zolotarev Y, Grachev S, Mikheeva I, Varlamov O, Zozulya A. Autistic children display elevated urine levels of bovine casomorphin-7 immunoreactivity. Peptides. 2014 Jun;56:68-71. Doi: 10.1016/j.peptides.2014.03.007. Epub 2014 Mar 20. PubMed PMID: 24657283.

[330] Addolorato G, De Lorenzi G, Abenavoli L, Leggio L, Capristo E, Gasbarrini G. Psychological support counselling improves gluten-free diet compliance in coeliac patients with affective disorders. Aliment Pharmacol Ther. 2004 Oct 1;20(7):777-82. PubMed PMID: 15379838.

[331] NEJM 357;17 Oct 25, 2007

[332] Ins Med Jour 38 (2008) 790-799

[333] Aliment Pharmacol Ther 2005;21:421-429

[334] Gut 2005;54:769-774

[335] Lichtwark IT, Newnham ED, Robinson SR, Shepherd SJ, Hosking P, Gibson PR, Yelland GW. Cognitive impairment in coeliac disease improves on a gluten-free diet and correlates with histological and serological indices of disease severity. Aliment Pharmacol Ther. 2014 Jul;40(2):160-70. doi: 10.1111/apt.12809. Epub 2014 May 28. PubMed PMID: 24889390.

[336] Serratrice J, Disdier P, Kaladjian A, Granel B, Azorin JM, Laugier R, Berenguer M, Weiller PJ. [Psychosis revealing a silent celiac disease in a young women with trisomy 21]. Presse Med. 2002 Oct 12;31(33):1551-3. French. PubMed PMID: 12422480.

[337] Liu X, Cao S, Zhang X. Modulation of Gut Microbiota-Brain Axis by Probiotics, Prebiotics, and Diet. J Agric Food Chem. 2015 Sep 16;63(36):7885-95. Doi: 10.1021/acs.jafc.5b02404. Epub 2015 Sep 1. Review. PubMed PMID: 26306709.

[338] Tjon JM, van Bergen J, Koning F. Celiac disease: how complicated can it get? Immunogenetics. 2010 Oct;62(10):641-51. doi: 10.1007/s00251-010-0465-9. Epub 2010 Jul 27. Review. PubMed PMID: 20661732; PubMed Central PMCID: PMC2944025.

[339] Bonamico M., Ferri M., et al. Serologic and genetic markers of celiac disease: A sequential study in the screening of first degree relatives. J. Pediatr. Gastroenterol. Nutr. 2006;42:150-154. doi: 10.1097/01.mpg.0000189337.08139.83.

340 Silvester JA, Weiten D, Graff LA, Walker JR, Duerksen DR. Living gluten-free: adherence, knowledge, lifestyle adaptations and feelings towards a gluten-free diet. J Hum Nutr Diet. 2016 Jun;29(3):374-82. doi: 10.1111/jhn.12316. Epub 2015 Apr 20. Pubmed PMID: 25891988.

341 Zarkadas M, Dubois S, MacIsaac K, Cantin I, Rashid M, Roberts KC, La Vieille S, Godefroy S, Pulido OM. Living with coeliac disease and a gluten-free diet: a Canadian perspective. J Hum Nutr Diet. 2013 Feb;26(1):10-23. doi: 10.1111/j.1365-277X.2012.01288.x. Epub 2012 Nov 15. PubMed PMID: 23157646.

342 Rose C, Howard R. Living with coeliac disease: a grounded theory study. J Hum Nutr Diet. 2014 Feb;27(1):30-40. doi: 10.1111/jhn.12062. Epub 2013 Mar 21. PubMed PMID: 23516989.

343 GRIEVE JW, PITT D. The coeliac syndrome. Med J Aust. 1948 May 22;1(21):660. PubMed PMID: 18866326.

344 N Engl J Med Oct.23 2003,1673-4

345 Proceedings of the Nutrition Society (2009), 68, 234–241

346 Clin Chem. 2007 Dec;53(12):2186-92

347 Previtali G, Licini L, D'Antiga L, Marseglia A, Ravasio R, Nembrini F, Greco S, Sonzogni A, Azzarà G, Ravelli P, Alessio MG. Celiac Disease Diagnosis Without Biopsy: Is a 10× ULN Antitransglutaminase Result Suitable for a Chemiluminescence Method? J Pediatr Gastroenterol Nutr. 2018 Apr;66(4):645-650. Doi: 10.1097/MPG.0000000000001773. PubMed PMID: 28991835.

349 Am J Gastroenterol. 2006,Mar;101(3):675-6.

350 Reddick BK, Crowell K, Fu B. Clinical inquiries: What blood tests help diagnose celiac disease? J Fam Pract. 2006 Dec;55(12):1088, 1090, 1093. Review. PubMed PMID: 17137549.

351 Valletta E, Fornaro M, Pecori S, Zanoni G. Selective immunoglobulin A deficiency and celiac disease: let's give serology a chance. J Investig Allergol Clin Immunol. 2011;21(3):242-4. PubMed PMID: 21548455.

352 Losowsky MS. A history of coeliac disease. Dig Dis. 2008;26(2):112-20. doi: 10.1159/000116768. Epub 2008 Apr 21. Review. PubMed PMID: 18431060.

353 Digestive and Liver Disease 39 (2007) 30-32

354 N Engl J Med Oct 23, 2003, 1673-4

355 MANSON G. NEGLECTED CHILDREN AND THE CELIAC SYNDROME. J Iowa Med Soc. 1964 May;54:228-34. PubMed PMID: 14143965.

356 choosemyplate.gov/MyPlate

357 Translated by Michael North, National Library of Medicine, 2002.

358 Green B. Use of the Hippocratic or other professional oaths in UK medical schools in 2017: practice, perception of benefit and principlism. BMC Res Notes. 2017 Dec 29;10(1):777. doi: 10.1186/s13104-017-3114-7. PubMed PMID: 29284529; PubMed Central PMCID: PMC5747024.

359 United European Gastroenterology Week When is a coeliac a coeliac? Report of a working group of the United European Gastroenterology Week in Amsterdam, 2001. Eur J Gastroenterol Hepatol 2001131123-1128.

360 Paul SP, Sandhu BK, Spray CH, Basude D, Ramani P. Evidence Supporting Serology-based Pathway for Diagnosing Celiac Disease in Asymptomatic Children From High-risk Groups. J Pediatr Gastroenterol Nutr. 2018 Apr;66(4):641-644. doi: 10.1097/MPG.0000000000001757. PubMed PMID: 28957985.

[361] Wolf J, Petroff D, Richter T, Auth MKH, Uhlig HH, Laass MW, Lauenstein P, Krahl A, Händel N, de Laffolie J, Hauer AC, Kehler T, Flemming G, Schmidt F, Rodrigues A, Hasenclever D, Mothes T. Validation of Antibody-Based Strategies for Diagnosis of Pediatric Celiac Disease Without Biopsy. Gastroenterology. 2017 Aug;153(2):410-419.e17. doi: 10.1053/j.gastro.2017.04.023. Epub 2017 Apr 28. PubMed PMID: 28461188.

[362] Bruzelius M, Liedholm LJ, Hellblom M. [Celiac disease can be associated with severe neurological symptoms. Analysis of gliadin antibodies should be considered in suspected cases]. Lakartidningen. 2001 Aug 22;98(34):3538-42. Review. Swedish. PubMed PMID: 11571796.

[363] Werkstetter KJ, Korponay-Szabó IR, Popp A, Villanacci V, Salemme M, Heilig G, Lillevang ST, Mearin ML, Ribes-Koninckx C, Thomas A, Troncone R, Filipiak B, Mäki M, Gyimesi J, Najafi M, Dolinšek J, Dydensborg Sander S, Auricchio R, Papadopoulou A, Vécsei A, Szitanyi P, Donat E, Nenna R, Alliet P, Penagini F, Garnier-Lengliné H, Castillejo G, Kurppa K, Shamir R, Hauer AC, Smets F, Corujeira S, van Winckel M, Buderus S, Chong S, Husby S, Koletzko S; ProCeDE study group. Accuracy in Diagnosis of Celiac Disease Without Biopsies in Clinical Practice. Gastroenterology. 2017 Oct;153(4):924-935. doi: 10.1053/j.gastro.2017.06.002. Epub 2017 Jun 15. PubMed PMID: 28624578.

[364] Trovato CM, Montuori M, Anania C, Barbato M, Vestri AR, Guida S, Oliva S, Mainiero F, Cucchiara S, Valitutti F. Are ESPGHAN "biopsy-sparing" guidelines for celiac disease also suitable for asymptomatic patients? Am J Gastroenterol. 2015 Oct;110(10):1485-9. doi: 10.1038/ajg.2015.285. Epub 2015 Sep 15. PubMed PMID: 26372508.

[365] Gidrewicz D, Potter K, Trevenen CL, Lyon M, Butzner JD. Evaluation of the ESPGHAN Celiac Guidelines in a North American Pediatric Population. Am J Gastroenterol. 2015 May;110(5):760-7. doi: 10.1038/ajg.2015.87. Epub 2015 Mar 31. PubMed PMID: 25823767.

[366] Previtali G, Licini L, D'Antiga L, Marseglia A, Ravasio R, Nembrini F, Greco S, Sonzogni A, Azzarà G, Ravelli P, Alessio MG. Celiac Disease Diagnosis Without Biopsy: Is a 10× ULN Antitransglutaminase Result Suitable for a Chemiluminescence Method? J Pediatr Gastroenterol Nutr. 2018 Apr;66(4):645-650. Doi: 10.1097/MPG.0000000000001773. PubMed PMID: 28991835.

+++++

Media/Interview Requests: JaquiKarr.com/contact

Printed in Canada

Library and Archives Canada

Author: Karr, Jaqui

Title: Your Brain on Gluten (It's Not Just Celiac Disease) Myths - Facts - Solutions

ISBN 978-0-9881303-7-1 Electronic Edition

ISBN 978-0-9881303-8-8 Paperback Edition

Publication date: First Edition, May 1, 2018

Medical Disclaimer: This book is strictly for information purposes. The author does not claim to diagnose or cure disease. The information provided is for the reader's information and as Ms. Karr suggests throughout the book, it is to be used in conjunction with medical help. Always seek a qualified professional for health issues.

Made in United States
Troutdale, OR
09/12/2023